Good and Powerful

Michael Yanuck MD PhD

Copyright © 2025 Michael Yanuck MD PhD

All rights reserved.

ISBN: 978-1-946600-43-1

DEDICATION

For Drs. Cami Zatkin and Gregg Kortz,
the extraordinary veterinarians who cared for Ini.

For Ini's friends, Beth Smaage and Caroline Mccaffrey,
who loved Ini and vice versa.

And for Ini's mom and grandma,
April and Doris.

Characters so often represent composites of several people, and happenings pertaining to one person ascribed to another that names have been changed, including my own. Although not always presented in the order they occurred, the events of this story are otherwise based on real events.

Love is Ini

She always wants me to be happy
She tells me so with every move of her body. Her warm brown
almond eyes gazing at me with trust and never ending interest.
Wiggly, Excited, fun .
Makes me laugh when she wants to go greet everyone with such
friendliness.
Making sure to take me on walks to the park to meet friends and chat
with the neighbors,
or to the river to be part of the change of seasons
To watch the wild turkey chicks grow from tiny to large,
To watch the start of plants grow in the spring, buds to flower! The
fruit to get big in the summer, ripening into sweet goodness,
The leaves to flare up in color before falling as the nights become
cold,
The sleepiness of winter when we dare to go where in the summer
the snakes roam, or we can see the river revealed by the bare trees.
Companion,
She always wants me to be near her
Excitingly, Wiggly greets me at the door at my return
She is quick to offer her Presence and a wet nose when I'm agitated,
upset, sad.
Comes and sits by me wherever I am.
Fills my heart with her quiet acceptance
Let's me stick my hand in her mouth to force a pill down her throat.
I know she will not bite.
Looks to me to see what I think we should do.
Will gently tug in the direction she wants to go.
Sick
Hard to watch her suffer
Hop on three legs
Post surgical pain
Loneliness of the recovery room with no ability to visit friends
Slowly re-introduce to walks, greatly improves the depression from
pain and loneliness.
Getting better day by day, but not full recovery.
We miss, do not understand, the sudden stabs of pain. She thinks she
is under attack! Whips her head back to see the danger! Nothing to
see! So she tries to run away from herself, but there is no running
away from yourself, now is there?
Cannot pee, some dribbles out of her on the bed. She is depressed.
The Bladder gets so full, can't walk, so much pain!

Finally Mom understands how sick She is, how much suffering she has.
Mom puts her trust in Doctor- please be right, help my fur baby get well 🐾❤️
Give me more time with my Ini.

CHAPTER ONE

Breaking the glass...

Our dog, Ini, is in the hospital.

The night before, I was listening to music (particularly, Steely Dan's Deacon Jones) while performing bioenergy with Ini and petting her. Given all that's going on with her (and the great source of unconditional love to me she's been her whole life) I just wanted to be good to her, honor her for all she's given me these years. She's brought so much joy to my life. Just her being here with me is such a comfort.

Even our cat, Cat Chow, seemed to sense something and hopped in bed with us.

Then, I experienced energy at my crown chakra, as Ini entered a deep state of sleep and undergoes a number of spontaneous muscular releases.

At around one in the morning, Ini indicated that she wanted to go out. That was not unusual, as she has been urinating with greater frequency; what was unusual was her anguished cries to come back in.

And when she did come back in, she jumped in my bed and, unlike essentially any other time, let me lay down beside her and stayed this way for hours.

Given all of this – the intense need to urinate every hour and change in behavior – that's the moment I decided I was 'shattering the glass and hitting the emergency button.'

I told Sara we had to take Ini to the emergency room to be evaluated in the morning and spent the rest of the night composing the following statement:

History of Present Illness
November 29, 2023

Ini's current symptoms and condition were first noticed by us about six weeks ago around October 14, 2023 when Ini demonstrated rather odd symptoms of increased urinary frequency that were not associated with displays of hesitation, pain or burning, as would be expected for a typical UTI.

Now, over the past days, Ini displayed such marked increased thirst and urinary frequency that we thought it necessary to bring Ini to the Emergency Department.

The second concerning issue is weight loss: During an appointment with Ini's oncologist, Dr. Moore, on November 1, 2023, she commented that although there was no evidence of cancer around Ini's recently excised anal mass, Ini had lost 4 lbs since her last visit (saying she went from 56 to 52 lbs.).

Ini has chronic pain from conditions including GME, TLPO and fracture, so we had previously thought that her weight loss might be helpful to take weight off her joints; however, after Dr. Moore's comment, we made a point of cooking for Ini and watching her eat substantially every day. Cooked items included ground beef, bison, chicken, fish, eggs. However, today we learned that Ini had apparently lost another 4lbs over the past month and is now down to 48 pounds.

Review of Ini's medical records indicate that her weight was essentially stable at about 63 lbs. before six months ago, and over the past six months, her weight has progressively decreased, as follows:

3/15/23	*28.5 kg*	*62.7lb*	*Bradshaw VCA*
5/25/23	*28.5 kg*	*62.7lb*	*MarQueen*
7/10/23	*27 kg*	*59.4lb*	*VCA Referral Center*
8/7/23	*27 kg*	*59.4lb*	*Bradshaw VCA*
10/14/23	*24.3 kg*	*53.5lb*	*Bradshaw VCA*
11/1/23	*23.3 kg*	*51.3lb*	*MarQueen*
11/16/23	*23 kg*	*50.6lb*	*Bradshaw VCA*
11/29/23	*22.1 kg*	*48.6lb*	*UCD*

Hence, 14 lbs. weight loss over six months; 11 lbs. over the past 4 months; 5 lbs. weight loss over six weeks; and 3 lbs. weight loss over the last 1 month (and this despite intensive feeding efforts over the last month).

Although this might suggest a 'wasting syndrome' like cancer, Ini had an abdominal CT performed on July 19, 2023 at VCA Referral Center, which was negative for evidence of malignancy.

Meanwhile, a general feeding pattern has developed, whereby Ini asks for food by indicating that she is hungry, but very soon after starting to eat, she stops and walks away from that food. Recently she has rejected a number of foods which were favorites, like freshly cooked human grade eggs, hamburger, grilled salmon, cod and chicken. Often, she communicates that she is still hungry and wants something else to eat, but can't seem to stomach eating more.

Furthermore, in the past weeks, it has felt like Ini has been trying to communicate something to me, but I don't understand what she is trying to communicate, and she responds with what seems like a combination of frustration, unhappiness, hurt and feeling dejected.

Other important elements of Ini's Past Medical History include the following:

1.   GME/ inflammatory meningitis-myelitis with spine pain and urinary retention, diagnosed in 2019 (following only partly successful R TLPO surgery); initially treated with Prednisone, but that had to be discontinued because of polydipsia side effect; currently treated with Cyclosporine...

CHAPTER TWO

What a difference a day makes...

At the Emergency Department at the UC Davis School of Veterinary Medicine, I received some hard looks from staff members who thought Ini's symptoms sounded mundane.

"What is this guy doing, bringing his dog to the emergency room for a common urinary tract infection?" they seemed to say.

But I was steadfast, and, over time, the veterinarians appeared to get it, although they were suspecting even worse than I was.

"It sounds like cancer," one said.

And then they found that not only did she have cancer, but it was a very aggressive form of urologic malignancy and her body was riddled with it (especially in her lungs), such that she probably had but a couple weeks to live.

Sara was especially hard hit, because when Ini underwent evaluations prior to a surgery for a couple of months ago (for suspected cancer) there were no signs of cancer in any of the imaging studies.

"In September, after Ini had been through a CAT scan and had surgery and then got discharged from oncology, I was in the euphoria of her having just been discharged from oncology," Sara confided to our veterinarian friend, Bubbles. "So, I was thinking, 'I don't have to worry anymore. Now, I can take Ini to be with my sister, and do this and that and have joy.'

"But Mike started telling me that there's something wrong," she continued. "Mike knew something, and I wasn't being serious about his concerns. And now she has this crazy fast-moving cancer going on."

Bubbles asked how I knew something was wrong? I said that beyond Ini's odd urination behavior, I was having these odd energy experiences, as well.

Okay, so what are 'energy experiences'? To answer that, I have to start somewhat from the beginning: Some thirty years ago, I was

Before the Innovation Accelerator project, or working with Kino engaged in cancer vaccine research at the National Institutes of Health (NIH), where my experiments ushered in an FDA-approval cancer vaccine and launched the new science of Neoantigen Tumor Immunotherapy. Then, I suffered a leg injury and conventional medical practices were not able to help me. So, I turned to alternative forms of healing and was pointed in the direction of Dr. Bruce Rind, who helped me and then trained in a technique called "bioenergy."

Bioenergy is an energy healing technique that the comes out of the osteopathic tradition. It's built on the principal that there is a human energy field, and in its normal state it flows in a regular, even pattern. However, when the body sustains trauma, blockages in the energetic circulation develop that can manifest in physical disease. Bioenergy, in turn, corrects those energy imbalances and awakens the body's innate capacity to heal. There's essentially no form of trauma that bioenergy can't attend; and performed with care, it has no harmful side effects or adverse reactions; it gives the body what it needs, when it needs it, at the exact dose required to facilitate healing.

To give you an idea about this approach, I'm going to offer this vignette about my first experience with it: On my first day of volunteering with Dr. Rind, he gave a cursory lecture on concepts in healing, then led me into a darkened exam room in which a female patient sat in obvious distress. Directing the woman to lay on her back on the examination table, Rind moved his hand above her body, then instructed me to do the same.

"Did you feel that?" he asked.

Oddly, I had felt something – like an energetic breeze blowing against my palm.

"What is this?" I asked.

"Bioenergy," he muttered under his breath.

"What's that?" I responded.

"It's the body's way of pinpointing a blockage," he said. "Energy gets stuck at the site of injury; it can't move, so it just collects there. Now feel for what direction it's going."

"How do I do that?" I inquired.

"Let the energy move your hand to whichever direction it wants to go," he instructed.

It moved my hand diagonally across her torso.

"That's right," he affirmed. "It's a stretch injury... Her body got wrenched against a seatbelt strap in an automobile accident. Now it needs to be corrected."

It's safe to say that I was utterly blown away, as a myriad of questions raced through my head: What was the source of this invisible energy? Why did it rise from the surface of the body? What information did it convey about the injury and source of trauma?

In due time I'd come to understand all these things, and then learn much more when difficulties I encountered with bioenergy led me to Qi Gong.

What is Qi Gong? In the words of my Qi Gong master, Master Chou, "Qi is the life force. The Universal Qi runs through all things. Trauma severs our connection with the life force. To restore the Gong, which can be translated as 'function', we have to remedy the source of trauma. This we do through the practice of Qi Gong. By ridding the body of trauma, we eliminate those things that stood in the way of our being fully natural. In this way, Qi Gong restores us to our true selves."

So, I was trained in Qi Gong. The ultimate in Qi Gong is Medical Qi Healing, which involves directing (or emitting) 'healing energy' at someone. With time (and the help of my friend, Sam), I acquired the skill to send healing energy.

So, finally getting back to Ini, I was trying to locate an energy disturbance/Qi blockage on Ini, but I really wasn't finding anything; instead, I had the odd feeling that I was sending healing energy (Qi emission), such that I was generating energy in my hand, which just didn't feel right?

"Something was blocked," Bubbles asserted.

More, it seemed there was something that required conventional diagnostics in order to determine (and, hence, was hiding from my ability to detect energetically), so to clue me in that Ini needed something else.

Hence, I'd brought Ini to the Emergency Department, and you know the result...

CHAPTER THREE

Condolences & Reflections...

My wise friend, Sam, passed along his condolences when I shared Ini's diagnosis.

"It sounds like you were expecting that, though," he asserted.

But I wasn't. It was my thought that her symptoms were related to some kidney issue that was perhaps treatable.

"I know you said you weren't," he responded. "But you knew there was something wrong.

"I was also hoping she wouldn't have cancer, but her appetite, weight loss and all that... Oh my goodness, I didn't want to say it, but... Oh, I feel so bad. How is she doing now?"

At the time she was lying on my bed, and I was playing music again as I pet her and performed bioenergy.

"Is she in any pain?" he asked.

The veterinarian had applied a fentanyl patch, so I was hopeful that that it was controlling her pain.

He again expressed his condolences.

"I have to say, though, even in her condition, because of all the love she gets, even with all the symptoms that are coming up, her demeanor and her character is really, really still peppy," Sam declared. "Especially when I go and I pull up in my car and she comes to me... It's amazing how she has such a wonderful character. She's a rare, rare dog."

Yes, 'bright and shiny', just like she was that first time I laid eyes on her.

I shared my disappointment – I'd laid out thousands of dollars before a surgery just a few months before to make sure that Ini didn't have advanced cancer before they took out an anal mass, because we didn't want to be doing a lot of wound care for a dog whose days were numbered.

And when that CT suggested the possibility of metastatic disease, I pointed that out to the veterinarian oncologist and suggested continuing to observe, but she assured me that what there was on CT was nothing and to go forward with the surgery.

"And you felt that the surgery wasn't going to do much?" Sam commented.

That's right. After all was said and done, there was no cancer ever found, and a cyst was all there ever was. Now, Ini's body is riddled with cancer, and this right after being discharged from care by the oncologist. How upsetting is that!

But, look, Ini is probably the victim of some oddball cancer of urethral origin that came out of the clear blue sky and rocketed all over her system – and that's that.

"I have to say that the cancer I've seen with friends and with relatives can all of a sudden be not there, and then all of a sudden be there," Sam responded. "Other times it's there and then it disappears. And you get everything in between that. So, it's so difficult to predict in cancer. And it's amazing when you hear about a cancer survivor, because nobody has a formula that says that you're going to survive. They always say, 'Well, we can do this procedure and there is this percentage of survival', but nothing is 100%, or even close to that.

"And, so, cancer itself is just one very mysterious illness in life. I've seen people survive, and I've seen people who you would think should survive all of the sudden rapidly decline.

"And, so, it's really, really difficult to pinpoint what the outcome will be for a patient. It's just very strange.

"I don't know if there's any hope, but will pray and consider whatever there is for Ini. Because all I know is that Ini is great, great dog..."

I confided that I was scared: Her lungs were riddled with cancer, and I was afraid I wasn't going to put her down in time to keep her from suffering.

"I think you'll know when the time comes," he responded. "When to make the move and all that. I don't think that you can plan for that. I think it's a gut level feeling.

"You know her better than anyone... And, anyway, I don't think Ini minds suffering a bit to be with you and April. It's just one of those things. She'll probably want to suffer and be with you until her suffering gets to a certain point that, by then, you'll know definitely."

I shared how it was that today while Ini was so drugged up, I was essentially ready to euthanize her, so she wouldn't really know it (that is, know what happened to her), but April wasn't ready.

"Ultimately, what matters is when Ini is ready," he asserted. "It has to be somewhere in between what you want, and what April wants, and when Ini is ready to let go."

"I tell you, Mike, death and dying has always intrigued me," he added. "When I was with people who were passing away, they knew when it was time for them to go. It would seem like, all of the sudden, a big burden would lift off of their shoulders and they lost the connection to life, and there was something they needed to go on to, whatever that is - whether it's an empty void or some type of regeneration or a heaven. Whatever? I've always felt that when the time comes, they're ready - They let go. And there's nothing that you can want to do to keep them here. They kind of reject that. It was that case for my mother, and for my grandfather long before that: All of the sudden, there is a quietness that speaks really loudly. Because that's how they become - Nothing mattered to them at that point. Things that were important to them were not important anymore.

"And that's where I think Ini will be. All of a sudden, even you and April will diminish in her mind, as she is ready to move on. Because, then, anything that's holding her to this world will be pretty much meaningless. That's what I've witnessed, even in my days in the hospital when I was an orderly taking care of terminal patients in college.

"Anyway, I think you'll know exactly what to do when the time comes."

He hesitated.

"Boy, it's really weird that we're talking about this, because I keep thinking of Ini as a very vibrant dog that just loves to live," he continued. "Loves to move around – But has this wonderful demeanor about her. She has this peacefulness all the time about what life is. And I think it's because you took such wonderful care of her that she has a beautiful outlook on life. I mean, for a dog, she seems to be quite at peace with being who she is."

I love who she is. I have always loved who she is.

"I mean, when she comes up to me, she's solid," he continued. "I mean, mentally. She doesn't bark. She's just, 'Yeah, I know who you are, because I know who I am.'"

Yes, and I know, too: She's a beautiful soul. I've always known that about her.

"So, she's very at ease," Sam commented. "And that's kind of neat. I've always had animals around me until the last few years; and all of these dogs, my goodness, they all have their wonderful personalities and such. And Ini is no exception. She's very unique in her aspects. They are all such characters..."

"It's too bad she won't be going with you to the East Coast," he continued. "She won't have that experience of moving out there with you."

I told Sam that I don't have feelings of "too bad this and too bad that." I just feel so blessed with what I have.

"That's the best way to look at it," he responded. "I was just thinking that she might have liked the snow."

Yes, she had always loved the snow.

Sam shared a story about one of his dogs experiencing snow for the first time.

"And it was kind of magical," he said. "Just watching how he was trying to deal with it."

Ini was essentially born and raised in snow. The first photo I took of her was in front of our Chamberlain house in the snow.

"Anyway, Mike, I'm sorry to hear this, but Ini had a good life," he concluded. "I know it's going to hit you so hard. Just always be comforted that she came into your life. She chose you..."

CHAPTER FOUR

Polite...

After Ini was discharged from the hospital, she peed so long that I think the only possible explanation was she hadn't urinated in the past two days (And this for a dog that had been peeing hour after hour at home).

I was sad that obviously she'd held her urine for those days, which must have been terribly uncomfortable.

But April was not surprised.

"She's so polite," she said. "She doesn't take food that isn't offered from your hand. She doesn't pee in the house..."

CHAPTER FIVE

Shock & awe...

Given how shocked April was at the diagnosis at UC Davis, she asked our regular veterinarian to confirm those findings by performing a repeat ultrasound on Ini at the clinic?

Although our veterinarian agreed, Ini wouldn't cooperate and refused to leave the car till it was too late.

Then, April asked a Vet tech about the fentanyl patch that had been applied to Ini and whether it was still properly attached? I didn't think there was any problem, so when the vet tech seemed to manipulate it, so to detach it from the skin, I got upset.

That's when April couldn't take it anymore and walked off to a nearby bench and hung her head and cried.

Meanwhile, I tried to re-establish the seal, but I wasn't able, and realized that I couldn't walk away from this and had to get a replacement.

So, I acquired a fentanyl patch at a nearby pharmacy, and, afterwards, the techs at the clinic kindly applied it (even with Ini still in the car), which gave Ini much relief.

They charged $45 for that.

Later, when we called a hospice service to inquire how much they'd charged for the same procedure, it was over $500...

CHAPTER SIX

Grateful for diabetes...

On the drive home, April made the point that it was probably the diabetes that led us to find the cancer; that is, she would not have been urinating hour on the hour without the diabetes.

"So that she suffered with uncontrolled diabetes for a while was not a good thing either," she said. "But without it we wouldn't have known about the cancer and had no idea that this terrible end was coming.

"I mean, it's awful that she suffered with the diabetes, but hopefully now she won't suffer a terrible end.

"I mean, with all due respect to Dr. Salkin [our regular vet], if she would have examined Ini, she probably would have stopped at the diabetes... She would have just said, 'Oh, your dog has diabetes. Here's some insulin. Take your dog home.'

"And Ini wouldn't have gotten the big-time pain medication - the fentanyl," April declared. "Ini would not have been this comfortable. It's letting her chase squirrels. She needed fentanyl."

Yes, we had taken Ini to the park and she had a good time and even chased the squirrels, which she had not done in the longest time.

"And this might make you want to reassess how you treat your patients," she concluded. "Because a CT is six months ago doesn't mean shit with these weird cancers..."

CHAPTER SEVEN

Like Ini?...

Even when we got home from the vet's, Ini was still too traumatized than to get out of the car.

As such, April spent the evening sleeping in the car with her.

Meanwhile, our cat, Cat Chow, laid down with me in bed, like Ini would. Laying on her side against my leg and accepting being stroked and petted, which were things she'd never done or tolerated before.

It was amazing – as though she were trying to be Ini for me – to help me, where I was so upset...

CHAPTER EIGHT

"... she loves Ini, too..."

Now, Cat Chow is usually the polar opposite of Ini. Where Ini is polite and sensitive, Cat Chow essentially does whatever she wants.

And if you don't let her do what she wants, when she wants... Well, there's going to be (as April would say) "punishment" and a hefty price to pay.

So, look, in the morning when I got up, Cat Chow was outside the door, wanting to get into the house.

The problem is, after Cat Chow gets in the house, she often wants out of the house... And I wanted to take a shower; and I live in fear that if I'm not available to let her out when she wants to, she's going to unleash the nuclear weapon – that which is my kryptonite; namely, cat pee.

So, I decided to keep her outside while I showered, with the thought in mind that I would let her in after my shower (and then be there to attend her wishes without disappointment).

However, when I got out of the shower, I found that not only was Cat Chow in the house, but she was in the bed with April and Ini (who had come in from the car while I was showering).

And this surprised me, because her usual morning pattern is to have some food and when she's done, leave the house.

But April wasn't surprised.

"She knows," she said. "And she loves Ini, too..."

CHAPTER NINE

Non-human accommodation?...

Where Ini was so sick (and April and I are so grief stricken), I called my medical provider and asked for a work excuse, saying I thought Ini needed and deserved my help right now.

But my provider told me she couldn't provide such an "accommodation" to care for a non-human ("Even if it is your soul-dog," she said) and suggested I reach out to my supervisor and request "personal" time-off.

Ini might be "non-human", but for 12 years she's been with me through thick and thin: Harrowing experiences like being caught in a white-out in the Northern Plains during a night when others on the Reservation froze to death. Through every blizzard, she's been there with me (and for me). She is intwined in my endorphin system. If there's someone else for whom you can make such an accommodation (other than Ini), my question is, Why?...

CHAPTER TEN

Walk to the park...

Getting up, it turned that more than food, Ini desired a walk.

I'd spent the three years of the pandemic in the park, studying to be board-certified in Addiction Medicine. It's something that usually takes a fellowship, but given my work with homeless Veterans (the vast majority of whom have problems of addiction), I was given the option of getting certified based on my experience and passing the Board. And the studying I did at the park with Ini. For essentially every hour that I studied, it felt like Ini was right there with me.

And the subject was intense, such that there were times in the park when I'd be feeling like it was hopeless, and I just wanted to go home, because there was just no way to learn all of this stuff on my own, and it was too much without a fellowship.

And Ini would be there urging me on, putting her foot (I mean, paw) down and seemingly saying, "Mike, I think you need to stay here longer and study some more. I think you can learn this as long as you're willing to put in a bit more time and effort."

So, I would stay at the park, and I would study under Ini's watchful gaze (that is, when she wasn't watching the squirrels).

And, lo and behold, I did pass the Addiction Medicine Boards. And that accomplishment might have not entirely been Ini's main motivation for getting me to stay and study at the park, it's not exaggeration to say that if hadn't been for those days in the park, I would not be a board-certified addictionologist with a planned appointment at Yale...

CHAPTER ELEVEN

Not my sled dog...

Nearing the park, Ini and I were passed by a fella on rollerblades being propelled by a couple of leashed and running German shepherds.

Watching, I wonder what it might have been like to be athletic and capable of feats like that?

Injuries early in life denied me a life of athleticism, and directed me, instead, towards scholarship, science and medicine.

And, thinking about it, I think Ini preferred it worked out this way.

Indeed, whenever I did do anything close to this fella on the rollerblades (like took my Onewheel on a walk with us, etc.), Ini never particularly appreciated it. She wanted to be able to enjoy the nature on our walks.

Hence, perhaps I could appreciate the experiences in my life (including the injuries), because I don't think Ini would have liked being tethered to a leash and effectively serving as my sled dog while I was on my rollerblades, declaring "Mush to the park" and "Take me here" and "Take me there."

I think my injuries have given her more an opportunity to 'smell the roses' and enjoy the path, and allowed her to be more who she is, rather than something I wanted to make her into...

CHAPTER TWELVE

Dogs as Medicine...

Meeting a neighbor at the park, he made the comment that
"dogs are medicine."

"They read our faces," he said, "and if they see we have negative
emotions, they figure out a way to help..."

It made me think about the other week when April, Ini and I
were downtown enjoying the fall foliage, and April came up with Ini's
"life goals."

She wants us to take care of her.
She wants to be with us.
She wants us to be happy.
She wants to go on a walk to the park
She wants to hang out with friends
And she wants not to be in pain. She wants to be healthy.

Why not these simple goals. What else good is there? Why want
anything else?

Indeed, at the time that April had offered these life goals, I'd
thought, "If everyone had those goals, it would be a much better
world - If all the nations of the world had those goals, it would be a
much better world."

Medicine for the world, I thought...

CHAPTER THIRTEEN

Lullaby...

It's interesting to me that despite how sick and weak Ini has become, she still feels an instinctual need to follow the routines that she's been used to: A walk to Caroline's in the morning; then a walk to the park; another walk to Caroline's in the afternoon, this time followed by visiting Lee & Linda and then Liza, before coming back by the levee, and then back to the house, before retiring with me to my room and laying at my feet on her dog bed as I work on my stories on the computer at my desk.

So even where April and I are willing to cater to her and do whatever she wants, it's the routine that she asks for.

Meanwhile (getting back to my evening routine), as I was dictating these passages at my desk, April commented about how it was that Ini was sleeping all through it.

"It must be like a lullaby for her," she said. "You talking to yourself. She's just so used to it. And it's just part of her daily schedule."

"And it's good," she asserted. "She likes being on a schedule. I think she's very peaceful here..."

CHAPTER FOURTEEN

Quantum Caring?...

Watching a *60 minutes* segment, they were talking about the new quantum computer, and when they got to the part with a medical expert talking about how this quantum computer was going to revolutionize healthcare, I turned the television off, because I was so disgusted.

I think the main problem when it comes to medicine isn't computer power, it's caring. That's what would make the biggest difference right now.

But, then again, Ini was being cared for, and going to doctors every week; being evaluated and reevaluated; and yet wound up with cancer too advanced for treatment right under their noses. Perhaps, a quantum computer would have made a difference – though I doubt it.

Because one thing for sure is, we're not going to cure death – At least, not the physical demise of the body. Death is going to happen to people and animals. People and animals are going to die. It is inevitable. It doesn't matter what kind of quantum computer we come up with where that's concerned.

Hence, I contend that what really matters, is, Are we going to figure out and prioritize treating each other with care?...

CHAPTER FIFTEEN

Underappreciated...

I've been unhappy to the point of disgust at the reaction of most of our acquaintances at the park to Ini's diagnosis. They've been blessed by Ini's love and attention for the past ten years; yet their responses are usually trite and limited to comments like, "Sorry," "Good luck," and "Oh, that's too bad. Hey, do you have an extra dog bag?"

Where I consider Ini such a wonderful member of the community they are about to lose, I found it shocking.

How can people be so superficial this way? I think. Who are these people who cannot honor Ini in a way I feel she deserves. Are these people incapable of things like that?

If there's a really upsetting part of this process, it's this feeling of guilt that I've wasted Ini's gift by putting her here where it wasn't appreciated.

Because, for me, Ini is like a guru, instructing me on how you can approach life with grace. How are you can be gentle and still get your point across with quiet humility, sensitivity, beauty and love.

It's been like having the Buddha in my presence. My own personal Jesus... Well, actually, that was someone else...

Then, April reminds me that where I have not always been sensitive to the loses (in dogs and other pets) of those at the park. Indeed, I have repeatedly been the recipient of the blessings and attention of other's pets and have not treated their loss by honoring them as they deserved. So, who am I to cast blame and doubt?

Everywhere in the world this is happening. We try to share what is great in life, and we are angry and disappointed when it is not appreciated.

And I imagine the deeper explanation for this is very personal and the source of a significant inner sadness...

CHAPTER SIXTEEN

Evolution & Endorphins...

I think, naturally, there's an evolutionary value and survival benefits to being in someone's endorphin system: It makes it so they're willing to be there for you through thick and thin. Because you have that biochemical connection and attachment. That love, so that you would be there for that person or creature, whereas others would not. Hence, where others don't have that attachment, you are willing to be the one to give when they need you. Support, nourishment, etc. That person will provide you needed help when there is essentially no one else who will provide that to you.

To this is the general fact that, as well as "personal love" involving endorphins, we also possess "greater love" that involves a higher caller for such things as to make things better in the world, which in my case involved such things as the development of cancer vaccine and then advancing Energy Medicine.

And the question we all face is balancing the different facets of our lives and loves: Sometimes, you prioritize the personal love, in which you honor those who are most important to you; Sometimes you focus on the greater love; and between the two, you just hope that you can get that balance right (though, for myself, I feel like I never do!)

But, as my father would say, "The best you can do is the best you can do..."

CHAPTER SEVENTEEN

Love and friendship in dreamworld...

Returning to the problem of Ini's terminal restlessness, it's just likes someone you love is saying to you, "Daddy, daddy, help me. I'm scared. I am so scared"; and you try to be as reassuring as you can be, yet it doesn't make any difference, because, it seems to me, it's something that the other person (i.e., Ini) has to come to terms with.

And when I try to fathom it, I wonder, What are we? Just these individuals of different species on this one little planet together for an infinitesimal amount of time where we'll ultimately just be swallowed up by the universe, so that all that really matters is the love that we have for each other.

The next thing I know, my friend Dino shows up at the house in his truck and we were smiling and talking, until I find I can't hear him because April is having trouble sleeping and breathing through her nose; so Dino gets out of the truck and meets me along the truck bed, so that we can hear each other better, and we were laughing about the whole thing together.

And then I awaken from the dream – The only thing that still lingers about it is April still having the difficulty breathing through her nose as she lay next to me.

So, there Dino and I were laughing about the things in this world over in dreamworld... And it just confirmed my feeling that the most important things are love and friendship – in this world and in the next world and probably every other one...

CHAPTER EIGHTEEN

'The neighborhood greeter.'

Telling April about the dream and my feeling that the answer to the riddle of how to make a difference in the universe is you just need to bring love and friendship into everything you do, she responded this way:

"That's what Ini does," she said. "Not always - Sometimes she gets angry when she has a strong reaction to something - But usually."

She reminded me what a woman on the trail said of Ini yesterday.

"She called Ini, 'The neighborhood greeter.' She was spot on. Ini is the neighborhood greeter. Not that many other dogs do that - Come right up to you and say hi."

Yes, that's always been Ini – From the first time I saw her as a pup, I thought, "Bright and shiny, and just loves people..."

CHAPTER NINETEEN

Terminal restlessness...

Ini is suffering from 'terminal restlessness', a relatively common symptom that afflicts cancer patients, such that during the night she is wide awake and unable to sleep.

Just like with people, I think the question of what's behind it, nobody knows for sure: The secretion of factors by the cancer cells affecting circadian rhythms? Or responses to the cancer? It could be any number of things.

And it makes caring for cancer patients notoriously difficult, forcing caregivers to stay up through the night with their agitated loved ones.

At about one in the morning, I took Ini for a walk and she ultimately came back in the house and settled down.

April and I talked about giving her meds to sedate her, but decided we wanted her to be herself during this time, and not doped up in any way, and if we could put some effort in and ride through this thing, then maybe we could give her that in these last few days...

CHAPTER TWENTY

Perfect Poop...

It's funny about things that are considered unpleasant and what might change that: I'd been worried about Ini, because she'd displaying continued signs of increased thirst and during the night, I caught her searching around in the backyard for water from stagnant sources, from which she might acquire infectious bacteria, food poisoning and diarrhea. So, I was very curious about her forthcoming bowel movement.

Then, arriving at the park the next day, Ini's steps quickened, as she turned the corner leading to her favorite place to poop.

As such, I began running, so to observe.

And lo and behold, it was a perfect poop; I don't think I'd ever been so happy about someone else's poop in my life.

I could have bronzed it...

CHAPTER TWENTY-ONE

Lo, great and honored spirit...

Today, April described how she and my mother-in-law, Doris, had taken Ini to the park, and Ini had engaged the younger, bigger, stronger dogs in play.

"I held her back in the end, because I didn't want her to hurt her shoulder," April said.

You did the right thing, I told her. It would have been terrible if Ini were now limping around in pain.

"But what if she's going off right now and that was her last rally?" she asked.

Then, it was great, I responded. She has something to look forward to in the next life - With a new body.

"But what if she's going off right now?" she asked. "Shouldn't we be holding her?"

I thought we should let her have some peace. She knows that we loved her.

Besides, she probably isn't going, unfortunately. Because it's not her heart that's the problem, but, rather, the rest of the body, that's riddled with cancer.

The other day Ini had woke up looking depressed and draggy, taking a long time before she got up, as though pondering the question, What's the point?

Later that morning, despite April and my willingness to cater her to whatever she wanted, she would partake in neither bison, nor chicken, nor fish, nor treats.

"You got a good gig here," April commented. "You sniffed those pants up [at the Sweat Lodge Ceremony at which she chose me] and you got a good gig. When you go across that veil, Ini, you go find yourself another good gig…"

I looked to Ini now and the following came to my head:

"Lo, great and honored spirit, Ini-She Who Brings Life, may the great spirit, Wakan Tanka, take you soon to the Happy Hunting Grounds…"

CHAPTER TWENTY-TWO

"She would just follow you..."

These days, Ini prefers to be outside on the porch, taking in the smells and sites of nature.

The nights have been relatively cold, though, and April has insisted that Ini come into the house when it gets late (even when covered in a blanket).

"Ini is so smart," she commented, as she came through the door after Ini. "Do you know what she did? She said to herself, 'Mom is going to make me go in, so I better go pee first.' So, that's what she did. She's so smart and so polite."

Yes, with that sweet nature, I thought. Just figuring out how to compromise and navigate the rules. There's just so much to learn from her.

"People talk about her being so well trained," April continued. "But we didn't train her. She just wants to cooperate. We don't need to figure out how to make her cooperate. She just wants to. Because she wants to please us."

Yes, I've always tried to respect her as a creature of the wild who offered me her companionship; and being that I wanted that companionship, it seemed only fair that I accept her as she was and not try to make her into anything she previously hadn't been or live in a way entirely different than she had been living.

Then, I remembered our times on the Northern Plains when we'd go walking for miles, enjoying the nature. We could be hundreds of yards apart, and, yet, when it was time to go home, all I had to do was call out to her, and she'd come back.

"You just reminded me of when she was a puppy," April interjected, "and I would watch you guys out of the window; and the snow was higher than she was, so she would hop... She would hop after you. And she would pop out into the air to manage the snow being too high. So that she would hop, hop, hop hop.

"And you would be far away, just walking. And she would be like hop, hop, hop, hop, hop after you.

"And you would just walk out into the wild, no leash, no nothing. She would just follow..."

CHAPTER TWENTY-THREE

Coyotes remembered...

"And the other thing I remember she would do," April continued. "She would be hunting. She would be walking alongside of you, but she would be hunting – Like, 'There's something there', and when there was snow, she would dive into the ground to find it."

I'd seen Ini do just that on the trail near the house.

"Maybe that's how she got the coyotes mad at her?" April commented. "She would go after their dens? And then they were done with it. They said, 'That one goes after our dens.'"

Yes, it might have been I saw Ini doing that 'diving' on the day that one very angry dark coyote chased her; Ini was running as fast as she could and whimpering when she passed me; and when I turned around, there was that black coyote coming after her.

I held up my hands and cried, "No, no, no", and the coyote veered off and broke off its attack.

But that coyote looked serious - Like it meant business.

April talked about a time when she had a standoff with a coyote that blocked her and Ini's way.

"I came down a trail and went to go its way," she said. "And it was like, 'No. Absolutely not.'"

"I think it was a mama coyote protecting its pups," she added. "So, I kind of did a stare off, but then I turned around.

"And Ini and me were walking, and that coyote followed us. We were escorted out..."

CHAPTER TWENTY-FOUR

Fentanyl & resistance...

April said of the fentanyl patch & Ini that "It's letting her be her."

In other words, it was bringing out the being inside who'd been so riddled with pain that she couldn't be that entity anymore.

Of interest, I spent the essentially the whole of the COVID-19 pandemic studying for the Addiction Medicine Boards with Ini at my side the whole time; and seeing how much the fentanyl patches have helped Ini has given me a whole new view and understanding for the enthusiasm that hospice doctors had for opioids in the 1990's, so to suggest their broader use, which, in many ways, lay as the origins of the Opioid Crisis.

And it's an interesting proposition that this same medication is at center of the current opioid crisis, responsible for the majority of the present overdose deaths.

So, I suppose it makes sense that it's been very difficult to get the medication: Yesterday, after collecting a refill fentanyl patch prescription at the vet clinic, when I went to the nearby pharmacy, I was told they didn't have fentanyl patches anymore. So, I tried to get the patches at a couple of different CVS pharmacies and (long story short) they told me they didn't carry fentanyl patches and it was up to the provider to find a pharmacy that did (This despite my insistence that that sounded like a very onerous task to be put on a provider.

In general, when it comes to this medication, everyone is making it a fight, so that trying to get it for my dying, cancer-riddle dog is coming up upon resistance...

CHAPTER TWENTY-FIVE

Retarded?

Taking Ini to the park, there was a mentally-handicapped young woman (who had long taken a liking to Ini) being escorted by two caregivers. And unlike her caregivers (who walked by Ini without a thought), this mentally-handicapped young woman was extremely attentive: Inquiring about Ini's weight loss; the fur that had been cut off everywhere; and the fentanyl patch on her ankle.

When I told her that Ini had diagnosed with advanced cancer, she empathized, telling me about a dog she had to put down in 2019 because of cancer, as well as a brother who she lost then; and sympathized, and treated Ini in a caring fashion, always making Ini the focus of attention.

And this was so much better than my interactions with neighborhood friends who, the other day when I told them about Ini's affliction, spent maybe a minute on that, and then took up many more minutes of Ini's limited time by telling me all about a recent trip!

What's wrong with people? Why don't they treat each other with care? Can't you see that I'm grieving and experiencing anticipatory loss! Even a mentally-handicapped person can see that. These are people with normal executive function. Yet it all seems to beg the question, Who are the ones who are actually mentally retarded...

CHAPTER TWENTY-SIX

Sacrifice?

I got mad at a friend this morning. He asked me if my mother-in-law (who'd been helping to care for Ini) had left and got back home in time for her granddaughter's 10th birthday party? When I responded that she was still here and I was grateful for it, my friend laid into me: Scolding me and declaring you can't put dogs ahead of people; telling me that turning ten was a really important mark in person's life and how I was contributed to traumatizing a child; and intimating what was a dog good for, except for pooping?

His words cut deep and wounded me. Reducing Ini to her bodily excretions brought me right back to the loveless and entirely utilitarian house of my father that I grew up in and never felt right to me.

And where children were concerned, there is a place to help them manifest a deeper love that goes beyond the superficial - And that's important at any age! And that helping people (even young people) understand there are priorities was important. That, of course your grandma want to be with you, but we're physical beings, so we can't be everywhere at once, and sometimes other people need us more and that doesn't mean they don't love you any less.

So, you provide reassurance and education in the hopes that your grandchildren wind up more than just superficial beings so that it's just "me me me" all the time; and also so that you (the grandmother) are more than some superficial wreck, only motivated by feelings of guilt and fear and, hence, arrive at living a full and deep life of love - for yourself and the others in your life.

I mean (for Christ sake!), all I ever hear from this granddaughter is how much she loves Ini! Well, how about if she shows it? And maybe more than just always talking about how much she loves Ini, she could act on it? And realize that Ini wasn't going to have any more birthdays, and that her grandmother was helping Ini, and maybe she'd want that more for Ini than her grandmother showing up at her birthday party? You know, accepts a sacrifice to help what she loves?

And my friend could give me a break, too? And respect that in this life I'd been granted a little piece of joy and happiness and source of unconditional love called Ini? And I hadn't had many gifts like that? So, maybe, you could let me honor that, even if it meant putting a dog ahead of a human once?

Postscript: Eagleman Story...

On the subject of 'sacrifice', my favorite Native American story from my years on the Reservations is the one about the eagleman? It began with a flood that caused such a deluge that only one person was left alive in the world – a single lonely woman. Soaring above, a giant eagle spots her and descends. Their eyes meet, and he tries to comfort her by taking her on his back and sharing with her that which is his greatest source of joy – the ability to fly. Surveying the world from up high, the woman glories at the wonder of flight. But returning to the ground, she again loses herself in grief for those she lost, and the eagle knows if she continues this way, she'll perish.

So, the eagle soars up to the heavens and pleads with the Creator to give this woman the gift of companionship with one of her own kind.

"This wish I will grant you," the Creator says. "But it must come with the sacrifice of that which you hold most dear."

The eagle accepts.

Not long after, the woman is surprised to see a man approaching.

And as he grows near, she can't help feeling like she's seen his eyes before...

CHAPTER TWENTY-SEVEN

The Stakes...

Ini's terminal restlessness continues to worsen.

As such, April talked about the importance of us working together to be there during the night to help Ini with her terminal restlessness.

"Because I think already we could have made a different decision," she said. "We can euthanize her any time. So, if we're choosing to keep her longer, then there are consequences for us and there are consequences for her. And if she's suffering at night so that we can have another day with her, then, to me, we have a moral obligation to be there for her while she's suffering.

"And I hate to give her gabapentin [pain medication], because even though it might help, it will dull her out during the day so that she can be herself – And, like, that's the whole point of it - So she can be herself.

"So, if we think that the terminal restlessness is too much, then it's just time..."

CHAPTER TWENTY-EIGHT

Moving to the next world...

As Ini slipped into a state of loss of consciousness, April asked me to tell her a story about Ini that I'd never told her, and she didn't know about, and only I knew?

I told April about how it was that five years ago when Ini was in the beginning stages of the GME, I felt the impulse to dance; I went to the summer concert series at that park at Zinfandel and Independence; and arriving there and looking into the crowd gathered around the band, I saw Ini's spirit there, joyfully filtering into the crowd, as though to say, "Yeah, Mike, I'm with you. I'm enjoying the dancing with you."

And looking to her now, somewhere between this life and the next, somewhere in dreamworld, I think, "Go to that world, Ini. Go to that place where there is no more pain. Where there's no more suffering. Where there's just joy. Go, go."

This deep sleep that Ini has entered looks like the same one that Ini has always been able to slip into from the very first time I of our encounter at the Sweat Lodge, when she lay down dead in the snow after I had pulled that last article of clothing out from under her, and she was ready to leave this life and go to the next if I didn't take her.

And then that time she crawled under the table after that larger dog broke her leg; entering that deep state of sleep, as those surrendering this life to go to the other... until April came and took her for care.

She could always go to that next place... It was always there, ready and waiting for her if we didn't embrace the gift - a gift from heaven, a gift from the spirits - she could always go back there.

"Even as Ini enters this deep slumber," April said, "she seems very comfortable with us."

Yes, that is a comfort: Me in front of Ini; April behind her; Ini going deeper and deeper into this place of slumber - place of peace - with those she shared her life with - those who love her most, and to whom have given her the most, and to whom she has most given.

Staring at her, I feel this sensation of breath blowing gently at my face. It's continuous and has no scent, so it doesn't seem like exhalation. It's more like air being fanned towards me, and I've never encountered or experienced anything like it before.

Can it be? Is this some energy coming at me? From her? Like some energy transfer? Some breath of life coming from Ini to me? Breath of life from she who brings life?

I have always wanted you. I wanted you from the beginning. I wanted you forever.

I never meant you any harm. I have made mistakes, but I have always loved you. You have given me a beautiful, wonderful, loving relationship.

Only love. You have given me only love.

If I have ever withheld a treat from you, it was only because I thought it was the right thing to do, because I was concerned about your diet or weight or G.I. tract. It was a decision based on care and love and trying to do what was best, even when I made mistakes...

As she sleeps this way, she's curled around me: my fingers at her heart; both her arms around my hand; her legs around my forearm; as though embracing the energy points that I've spent a lifetime sharing with others to make bioenergy tangible to them; now she's embracing those points. Perhaps perceiving energy from those points? Energy that's probably moving from me to her, and from her to me; and I'm still feeling energy teeming at my crown chakra. My lovely, wonderful soul dog. Moving to the next world. Sharing the experience with me...

CHAPTER TWENTY-NINE

"Something new..."

April said that Ini had a different energy to herself today; whereas yesterday she was letting herself go deep into the sights and sounds of the animal world and chasing squirrels, today it was different.

I'd like to think it was because we gave her her fill of the animal world yesterday, like when she all but got a squirrel.

"She caught that squirrel," April declared, tearfully. "She could have had it, but she let it be. Everybody knows that."

It was just like that day with the baby deer: Following that day I described in my book, *She Who Brings Life*, when she went prancing in the forest with that baby deer, and, after, seemingly had her fill of chasing deer, and was ready for something new, like leaving the Reservation for IHS Headquarters.

I'd like to think that yesterday we helped give her her fill of the wonderful things in nature to be found in this life - This world.

And now she's again ready for something new...

CHAPTER THIRTY

"No fixing it..."

After a day of Ini growing weaker (so that she was having difficulty standing) and considering euthanasia, Ini applied what little energy she had left to direct me to let her out of the house through the garage door, then went to the back of the car and stopped.

"Where do you want to go now, sweetheart?" I asked. "Where do you want to go now?..."

Later in the night, I awakened from sleep to the realization that by going to the car, Ini was telling me it was time to go to the hospital.

"That's what we've done whenever she needed to get fixed," April commented. "When she needed to be medically fixed, we got in the car."

But there was no fixing this problem, and stuck in my logical mind, I hadn't felt for what my doggie was trying to say.

What must she be feeling? I thought. Did she feel unheard and uncared for? Like I didn't understand she had a problem? Or, if I did, that I didn't want to help her?

Then, as I lay feeling so upset at myself for not listening and not understanding her, Ini rolled on her back – Her way of calling me to take a little break from what I'm doing to enjoy a bonding interaction between us.

Hence, in spite of my failures, she still reaches out to me and doesn't turn her back on me...

CHAPTER THIRTY-ONE

Surprising psychological journey...

On the subject of scheduling Ini's euthanasia or not, April posed the following question:

"What would leave you with more trauma? – [1] A decision to hand her over to someone who kills her, with the intention of preventing her from further suffering? [2] Waiting until she has that suffering and then [euthanizing]? What would be more traumatic?"

This question took me on a surprising psychological journey:

In college I had a summer relationship which was one of pure bliss; but I cut it short because I felt the need to get back to my usual intensive studying. In this way I gave that relationship an unnatural end - and it's been a source of pain ever since; And now I think that one of the reasons I want to hang onto Ini for every minute that I can, is because the relationship with her has been pure bliss, and I'm trying to make up for my previous mistake.

This I consider the greatest source of personal failing in my life: I had unnaturally ended that relationship in college; it didn't have to die - I killed it; and I've been hurting over it ever since.

And what was the lesson learned from that experience? - Don't unnaturally end a relationship. And (in this circumstance) it was translating into a desire to not unnaturally end Ini's life, but, rather, see her through a natural death (Though not one that included any sort of intense suffering, but, rather, just to the moment that it was clear she truly wasn't enjoying her time on this planet anymore).

Nevertheless, the unearthing of the college experience made it clear to me that in doing what I did back then, I had effectively plunged a dagger into my own heart; and for the past twelve years I think (to a certain extent) Ini has been plugging that place of hemorrhage; and, now, sooner or later, that plug has to come out.

April countered that in those moments of clarity, Ini was experiencing sparks of real joy.

"And her mind is all there," she said.

"And her heart is there," my mother-in-law echoed.

Still, she was only getting worse, I responded. Why not avoid any suffering?

"But would that leave you with extreme trauma?" April asked. "A trauma that you would take into the rest of your life?"

"I mean we are blessed with the fact that the Referral Center is just five minutes away. If any terrible thing happened to her, she probably won't suffer it for more than an hour.

"So, what would leave you with more trauma? Or suffer because we couldn't make a decision? All the veterinarians are telling us that euthanasia is the best thing for her. She had to make the decision to kill her before this terrible thing happens to her. So, we're walking away knowing that we kept her from having this thing before. But if we didn't, we could have some more time with her in her body. What would be more traumatic?"

Yes, in some ways all this did speak to something that was very personally traumatic to me.

In college I had a relationship which was one of pure bliss. And I cut it short. I walked away from it before it's time. I gave it an unnatural end. And it's been a source of pain ever since. and now I think that one of the reasons I want to hang onto Ini for so long, for every minute that I can, it's because the relationship with her had been pure bliss. And I'm trying to make up for a mistake.

"Then, again, what would be the more traumatic thing for you? A decision to hand her over to someone who kills her with the intention of preventing her from further suffering, versus waiting until she has that suffering and then limiting the amount of time that she's suffering? What would be more traumatic?"

"I think it's a question for me, too, and maybe we should sleep on it," she concluded...

Overnight, I considered the long-term effects of that relationship in college...

When I killed the relationship with you, I drove a dagger into my own heart.

It would have long range implications.

I became a Flying Dutchman when it came to relationships after that. I was not open to love others tenderly...

April had called Ini the glue holding us together.
She couldn't be more right...

Postscript:

It happened that the following day, that person from my college relationship, 'Bubbles', called me out of the blue.

"I just had a feeling like I should call you," she said.

She's a veterinarian, and when I told her about Ini and her seeming willingness to endure suffering to be with us, she commented of pets in general, "They live for us."

Based on the experiences that follow, I think she's right...

CHAPTER THIRTY-TWO

Choosing a gift...

Ini is in another deep state of slumber.

April wondered that some internal pain is responsible for triggering Ini's deep, dissociative states? States in which Ini would just let go of everything... Let go of life. The way she did that first night that I encountered her at the sweat lodge ceremony, when it seemed like if I didn't take her home after pulling out that last article of clothing from under her, she was going to die right there in the snow.

Or the time when her leg was broken by that larger dog, and she crawled under the table, like she'd given up on all hope.

The source of the first might have been psychic pain? The second physical pain?

What they have in common is a certain surrender. A dissociative state that is associated with a willingness to let go of life.

But whereas there was a remedy for those previous situations, there wasn't one this time: This time, it can't be remedied with a home to go to. Or the setting of a broken bone. I can't undo the cancer. This time I can't help her. This time April can't help her. She has to rely on something else to help her. The great spirit. God. It's just the way life is.

I think, "All life long, she'd been able to enter these deep slumbers – in some dreamspace between this world and the next. The time at the sweat lodge ceremony where she chose me... I didn't have to invite Ini in; I could have left her lying in the snow, and she would have perhaps been just like she is here.

46

And April didn't have to come to the Reservation when I called after Ini's leg was broken to bring her to the Veterinarians to set it… We could have left her right under that table, and again she would've been just like she is here.

At any time following the diagnosis of the cancer, we could have taken the veterinarians' advice and euthanized her, and again she would have been just like she is here.

She could always just move to the next world: If her gift wasn't recognized in this world, so be it - it's our/their loss… She moves to the next world.

But choosing to be with her in all of these circumstances was an opportunity to embrace this great gift of love that has blessed us for a lifetime.

And I become aware that in this moment, I am standing straighter than I ever have in my entire life.

It's like what that speech teacher told me in undergraduate: that one day I was going to be so free and relaxed, but not only with my shoulder no longer be hunched and my head jutted forward, but my head would be hanging so far back that it would be behind me.

I could do that right now.

When I invite my life to be full of joy.

When I invite Ini to fill me with a breath of life...

CHAPTER THIRTY-THREE

Breath of life...

And perhaps I could be like Ini? Bright and shiny like she is? Just go out there into the world and be love?

If someone latches on to you, then that's their good luck.

If they don't, just move to the next world.

Live life sharing your gift. Sharing love.

That's the commonality between me and Ini? That's how we're similar? I recognized a kindred spirit when I saw Ini. I recognized it from the beginning.

And considering these things, there's something really tremendously different that's happening in my own body: my chest is tremendously opened. I am sticking it way out in front of me. Like I never have before. It's wide open. The energy beaming at the top of my head just confirms the connection. My stance feels normal and even, grounded and balanced.

Like I've truly been given the breath of life.

From she who brings life...

CHAPTER THIRTY-FOUR

Scouting out the next place...

And lo and behold, with a stretch, Ini is back. She came back to us. From some dreamland. From some other place. From being right at that veil between life and death. She came back to us.

"She's scouting out the next place," April said, eyes filled with tears of joy.

I kissed her and got close to her again; I'd been too afraid to get close while she was in that altered state, for fear it would be too much for me should she slip away in that moment.

But the moment she came back, I brought her close enough to me, and enjoyed that puppy scent that I love.

It's so wonderful, I thought. To have her back...

CHAPTER THIRTY-FIVE

Puppy pile...

Ini comes into bed with April and me, and lays down in between us, with her back such that my legs are literally pushed off the bed.

"That's something that Ini never got in this life," April said. "How to make room for everybody in the bed."

But it's a funny thing: At that moment I had been thinking about how I longed for the experience of being in a puppy pile with her, all squished together.

And, in that way, Ini did just the right thing...

CHAPTER THIRTY-SIX

Ini kind of day...

April took Ini for a walk around the park, where they met Dino and Marge, and Higgins and Glenn, and also Ingrid and her dogs.

"And they all spent good time with her," April said. "They all hugged her and interacted with her and talked to her and gave her treats.

"And she had a long time with Caroline.

"It was an Ini kind of day."

April commented that it wasn't going to be the same on Thursday, when April had made an appointment for Ini with the oncologist to get a second opinion.

"She's gonna be like, 'Oh, mom, do you really need to put me through that.'

"And I'm like, 'Yes, honey, if I'm going to kill you, I need to know for sure.'"

Then, April became tearful and cried...

CHAPTER THIRTY-SEVEN

Ini comforting us...

Personally, I didn't think the second opinion made sense: Ini was disintegrating before our eyes – with less appetite, less consumption of food, more pain, more fatigue, more restlessness, etc.

And, here, April was telling me she doesn't want Ini to suffer, and asking over and over again, "Should we just euthanize her?"

But April felt Ini was willing to do this for her.

"Ini came to you when you needed comforting," she said. "She went out of her way to cuddle up to you, in spite of everything that she was going through with that bloody diarrhea and as sick as she was feeling."

Here, she was alluding to the other day when the Emergency Department veterinarian literally told us not to bring Ini there anymore, because she was too complicated and sick for them to care for, and when we returned home, I took to bed, because I was so upset.

"So, I think she'll do the same for me," April concluded...

CHAPTER THIRTY-EIGHT

A gentle way...

April asked what I wanted for Ini?

I said a gentle goodbye and not a lot of tears; that I felt strongly that I would see Ini again in the spirit world, and a "see you later until then" was what I wanted, as opposed to a lot of emoting.

April got upset.

"You can't tell me not to cry during this time."

I'm not telling you what to do, I responded. You asked me what I would like and I was simply saying.

At which time, Ini promptly got up from where she was lying next to the garage by the car, and did what she usually does when April and I argue... Went to someplace else.

Which had the effect that it always had: To make me disengage, and go to Ini and comfort her and apologize for my negative energy; that I should have done better and owed her more than that in her time of need...

CHAPTER THIRTY-NINE

The Great Mystery...

April performed DNA testing on Ini, saying she wanted to "try to unravel the mystery of who her parents were before we were her parents."

I say Ini's parents were God and Wakan Tanka before we were...

CHAPTER FORTY

"She wants to be with us..."

Ini has taken to wanting to spend her hours outside, especially on the front porch near the mulberry tree with its beautiful yellow falling leaves.

April talked about bringing Ini inside last night.

"I got cold and tired and was falling asleep in the chair," she said. "So that I was finding myself leaning off the chair and needing to lie down.

"And it broke me that I couldn't stay out there," April continued, "but I was falling asleep on the chair.

"And Ini did not want to come in. She was begging to stay outside.

"But I couldn't take it outside anymore.

"So, I tried to get her to come in... She didn't want to. She stayed, looking at me and begging me to stay out there.

"And then she realized I wasn't coming back out, so she got up.

"But, first, she went and peed before she came in."

Always polite, I thought.

"She could have persisted. She could have put her foot down and said, 'I'm not coming in until you carry me in.'

I think Ini accepts our weaknesses. I think she always has.

Like April has said, Ini has always wanted to please us.

"She wants to be with us," April said...

CHAPTER FORTY-ONE

"Cold and dark..."

Following coming inside, Ini made several attempts to get up from her dog bed and follow me into the kitchen, but wasn't able.

I feared she wasn't going to be able to get up after this – She was too weak.

"She ate two plates at midnight," April said in response. "You don't think that's going to make a difference?"

I didn't think so - The cancer was just eating her alive.

"Should we take her back outside, so that she could enjoy the sights and sounds out there?"

It was two in the morning and near freezing out there, so that I thought it was too cold for us.

"I have to tell you," she began. "You know how I told you a few days ago that I was mad at you for letting her outside in the cold and the dark? But she's proven to me that that's where she wants to be. So, it makes me not feel so bad that she'll be out in the cold and dark, because she likes it. She likes being out in the cold and dark."

She always has. It was a cold and dark night that night she chose me - A creature of the wild who decided to gift herself to us.

"You're so amazing, Ini," April said. "Can I give you some warmth for just a little bit?..."

CHAPTER FORTY-TWO

Going round in circles...

April again lamented about bringing Ini inside.

"I wasn't thinking," she said. "I could've brought out the sleeping bag."

Yes, just like I wasn't thinking when she approached me about getting in the car. I guess we're both a little out of our minds with what's happening and this whole euthanasia decision that's facing us. We can't even see what's right there in front of us.

April asked if I wanted to put Ini in the car and take her to the hospital?

I said I wanted to do what Ini wanted; I felt as though last night I had effectively told her there's no going to the hospital for this - Because there's no fixing this.

And yet she opened herself to me, employing me to come and be with her by rolling on her back, which had always been her signal for me to do that. And it was as though she were saying, "In spite of you not getting me help (and I don't know why you didn't?), I am not turning my back on you."

She was still willing to open herself to me. She was still willing to bestow upon me her gifts of love. And if that was the case, then I wanted to be the recipient of that for as long as possible.

Maybe it would have been easy to go to the hospital when she had asked? Maybe I could have convinced myself that even though it wasn't fixing things the way it ever happened before (i.e., fixing things to promote life), it was still fixing the situation, and I could delude myself to want that.

And maybe it wasn't a total trick and betrayal. Maybe this was the kind of fixing that Ini wanted, too? Even if it were different than any other reason that I'd ever taken her to the hospital?

She was suffering from a condition, and this was the treatment.

But the outcome would be different; instead of coming home to me more well, she would not.

In this way, at least I had not led her to a different outcome than she was expecting.

Now, if it were at all possible for her to be with me until she was no more, then I wanted that.

At the moment she indicated that she was in significant pain and suffering, I would end this.

But before that, I didn't want some stranger to just take her away from me - No matter the caring intention.

"What all the different veterinarians have said to me," April inserted, "is, 'We can make it so she doesn't suffer. Why wait until she suffers? You can make it be no suffering.'"

Because she has spent her life (or at least a good part of it) suffering in order to be with us. Somehow it seems that it has been worthwhile to her to endure the pain of life in order to do that. And if she is willing to endure suffering to continue to be with us, I feel like then I wanted to give her that opportunity.

April described all of the terrible things that she'd been told could possibly happen to Ini.

"I was told she could start having seizures and she could start crying. It could add to the trauma for us and for her.

"And that when she's suffering, death is the kindest option."

She reflected about her grandmother.

"Was that a good death?... When she just slipped away?"

Perhaps for her it was (though for April, it was traumatizing).

"Because now that I'm hearing about all these other ways, and she slipped away so peacefully."

Yes, when the cancer vaccine I spearheaded was approved for FDA-clinical trials, the doctor engaged in those trials once told me that, no matter how much money people have, most "die like dogs."

"What did he mean?" she asked.

He meant it's unpleasant. Most nobody wants to die. You don't really know what's out there. What you do know is that you're not going to be here anymore. Here is the only place that you can really be sure of. Seems to me it's an individual decision what you'll suffer to be with those your love. God knows I watch that for a year with Ethel, enduring the worst pain known to medicine to be around for those she loved.

"Why is she so weak?" April asked of Ini.

Among other reasons, it's because the cancer is eating her. It's just what cancer does.

"What if we feed her something? I would have given her more, but I was afraid she would have a tummy ache."

She shook her head.

"I'm going to be really hard on myself for years probably that I didn't stay out with her," she lamented.

And should I be really hard on myself for years that I didn't recognize that she wanted to get in that car and go to the hospital?

"But even if you had been able to do that, all you would have been able to tell her is, 'It's not going to hurt.'"

I stepped back.

I hadn't even thought about that, I responded.

In any event, if there was one thing I knew for certain, it was that I couldn't imagine Ini wanting either of us to be suffering for years over anything.

"Can we open up the glass door and give her some of the sights and sounds of the outside?" April asked. "She so wants to be outside. Where she's suffering, at least she can smell and hear the outside. And you can be warm and put on your coat and wear your thermals and put on your ski pants."

Yes, I said...

CHAPTER FORTY-THREE

Ini at the Sweat Lodge...

Some of you know that ten years ago, I began writing about Ini. What follows is the first story about Ini...

On a cold winter night, the temperature well below zero, those inside the sweat lodge crawled out through the canvas flap into the elements. I was among the last to leave. The others having formed a line, I shook hands with each.

"Mitakuye Oyasin [We are all related]," we exchanged. "Mitakuye Oyasin."

Coming to tribal elder, Orville White Buffalo, he held my hand in both of his.

"Doctor, I'm sorry to hear about your wife," he said.

I nodded. I'd shared that we'd been having difficulty conceiving a child.

"I prayed for her," he continued. "I think we all did."

The line dispersed. Crossing the jagged, frozen snow, I reached down to where my clothes lay. But instead of clothing, my hand encountered something small and naked, like an infant?!

Assuming it must be a wild animal, I sprang back, hoping whatever it was would do the same. But, to my surprise, it didn't, and instead emitted a chorus of sweet, sorrowful moans. Attempting to make out the identity of the creature, I narrowed my eyes. But there wasn't enough light. I looked to the heavens; it was a moonless night with an odd belt-like river of stars that stretched from one end of the horizon all the way to the other.

The Milky Way? I thought.

But even under the light of all the stars in the galaxy, the creature remained a mystery, shrouded in darkness.

Then, from the embers of the fire pit used to heat the ceremonial stones came a sudden 'crack', and the corresponding burst of light gave form to the creature.

It's a dog, I thought. A puppy.

I reached down and caressed its soft fur; but this seemed of little reassurance to the small animal, as it continued to whimper.

"Did someone lose a dog?" I called out. "There's a puppy here."

From around the ceremonial grounds sprang a chorus of good-natured naysaying.

"Not my dog, Dr. Mike," one said.

"Not my dog," said another.

"You better take that dog, Doc," said a third, "or else it's going to wind up in the soup."

In the general laughter that followed, I worked determinedly to extract my clothes out from under it.

With each article of clothing I removed, I expected the little thing to get to its feet and scurry off.

But it remained.

Finally, removing the last of my clothing, the animal fell back in the frozen snow, belly up, motionless and silent.

Rising to a stand, the little creature was swallowed up in the darkness created by the space between us. I gazed in the direction of the gate. The others had left and the grounds were silent.

I could leave, too, I thought. There was nothing to stop me – No one to tell me otherwise.

Then I thought, What about a little piece of joy for me in life? Why not? Why not a little piece of joy for me?

And acting on that spontaneous impulse, I bent low and wrapped the pup in my towel, then tucked it under my arm and whisked it away to my car; the pup offering no resistance, as its weight sank contentedly into my hand...

CHAPTER FORTY-FOUR

Source of void?...

   Inside, Ini seemed to be more at peace with me. Leaving her with April, though, it seemed I was coming back to find her anxiously sitting up and looking at me; whereas when I stayed (and April went off) that wasn't happening.

   Laying down, I fell asleep next to Ini, but awoke to a feeling of being in some vast dark, empty void in space and it scared me that Ini might be going into such a void?!

   Where did this come from? I thought. Am I forgetting my own experience? This isn't my spirituality. Mine is based on that flash of white light coming from Elizabeth at that moment that she went to some otherworldly place.

   That's where my dog is going. Where did this 'void' thought come from?...

CHAPTER FORTY-FIVE

Source of spiritual belief...

What follows is the experience that lay at the core of my spiritual beliefs.

At the peak of my success with the cancer vaccine, I can still remember where I was when the thought crossed my mind, "Okay, let's say we are able to cure cancer. What then? People are still going to die. How are we going to cure death?" And to this I believed there was no answer.

It wasn't long after I had these thoughts that my leg injury occurred, then my path to bioenergy, and, ultimately, an answer to my question.

It happened at my friend Wah's house: He, Elizabeth and I would get together on the weekends to practice Chi Gong in his basement; but on this occasion, I was tired, so when the two of them got up to practice, I told them to go on without me.

Then, just as they were about to start, Elizabeth turned and said, 'Mike, watch my aura.'

I'd had a couple experiences seeing auras, and said I would, then sat back on the couch.

They began to practice, and – sure enough – I saw Liz's aura. It looked like this thick film of buzzy gray stuff coming off all around her.

In turn, she was patting herself, starting at her head, to her shoulders, then torso, and this gray film seems to be moving down into the ground.

'Good,' I thought, watching. 'She's probably getting rid of a lot of bad energy – turbid chi. I bet she's going to feel a lot better after this.'

Then - out of nowhere - there's this burst of white light that flashed from her! Just for a second - Bang! - like a firefly or quick explosion!

I jumped back on the couch, thinking, 'Whoa! What was that?!'

Meanwhile, Elizabeth was trembling all over. She motioned with her hands, too terrified to speak. She told me to hold her - Wah, too – saying she felt cold and seen something that scared her.

Then, she told us her vision: She saw herself carrying a dead body from a past life to a lot of otherworldly, happy-go-lucky creatures that took the body, then told her to go back to her life.

From this experience – between what I saw and what Elizabeth described – I derive my spirituality – An unwavering, unshakable belief that, at its core, life was about a spirit entity learning the lessons of the universe on a physical plane...

CHAPTER FORTY-SIX

Real dog...

"Still want a toy dog?" April asked.

She was referring to my childhood and an experience at the thrift store where we lived in South Dakota that I'd documented in my earlier book about Ini, *She Who Brings Life:*

As the weeks past, life settled into a predictable routine. On Saturday mornings I went into town for coffee and to buy Ini a fifty-cent stuffed animal at the church-sponsored thrift store. Entering the thrift store this week, my eyes gravitated to a jigsaw puzzle in the window display, the pieces coming together to produce a puppy whose expression and coloring was not unlike Ini's, and I was reminded of the puzzles April used to put together while I was away looking for jobs.

"So, you like puzzles!" the clerk said at the checkout counter. "When I was a little girl, I used to love doing puzzles. I'd do the simple puzzles, like this one here. I'd do them over and over. Then, my mother insisted that I do more 'age appropriate' puzzles. I found them really difficult and frustrating and they lost all enjoyment for me. So, I stopped doing them."

I smiled, as her story had rekindled a memory from my childhood.

"When I was maybe twelve," I said, "I received some money from my grandparents for my birthday. When my mom asked what I wanted to do with the money, I said I wanted a mechanical toy dog."

I shook my head.

"Can you imagine?" I asked. "What 12-year-old boy wants a mechanical toy dog for his birthday?"

"Did you have a dog?" she asked.

I shook my head.

No, I responded.

Then, it occurred to me that I'd been mistaken and I had had a dog: His name was Blackie – probably a black Labrador-German shepherd mix. He was just a puppy when my mom brought him home in a paper sack. She got him from a friend who found him wandering the condominium complex. I could still remember how he looked that night: Sweet, embarrassed, nervous, scared. From the day on, he was my dog.

And that dog could do anything: Play soccor, frisbee, fetch. The only time he ever whined was when his neck got caught in the tetherball rope – My father was still with us then, because I remember it was he who went outside and untangled Blackie.

After my parents divorced, we moved to another house. The house didn't have a fenced-in backyard. I guess my mom hadn't thought about it before settling on the place. She didn't know how to do a lot of things. I guess she kind of relied on my dad for that. We chained the dog to a tree. I don't think Blackie liked that. He kept on getting tangled in the chain – wrapping it around and around the tree till he wound up stuck there.

And there was this small dog named Foxie. It belonged to our next-door neighbor. They would let it run free and it would come around into our backyard. I don't think it meant to tease Blackie – maybe, it did.

One night Blackie broke the chain and went after Foxie. It was just my younger brother and me that night (I don't know where my mother was). I went after Blackie and caught her across the street. I was pulling Blackie back to the house when he lounged and broke free. This time, he bit Foxie and shook her, tearing the skin. I grabbed Blackie, and my brother took Foxie. I'll never forget the sight of my brother's shirt, full of blood.

When my mom got home, we took Foxie to the vet and got her sewed up.

Returning to the house, my mother made some calls. Afterwards, she told me that Blackie had to go to the pound and we couldn't keep him anymore.

Blackie was locked in the bathroom. I went inside and stayed with him through the night. He was as gentle as he'd ever been. Nothing to be afraid of. Looking the same as he did when he was a puppy. Embarrassed. Scared.

The following day I went to school and spent the whole time crying. Classmates came by and asked, What's the matter? But when I told them, they didn't understand...

"So, you wanted a mechanical dog," the clerk reasoned, "that no one could ever take away."

Smiling, I nodded approvingly – She had solved the puzzle!

"Do you have a dog now?" she inquired.

Yes, I said. Her name is Ini...

Back in the present, I told April, no, I wanted my real dog.

"And this is a real dog," she responded. "This is like the ancestral dog."

Gift from the spirits...

CHAPTER FORTY-SEVEN

Unable...

During the night Ini experienced her usual anxiety and agitation, likely as pertains to the terminal restlessness. I wanted to hold her and put my arms around her, but there wasn't space for that, as her back was flush against the sliding glass door.

Over time, she continued to get more agitated, and, using her upper limbs, she attempted to pull herself up, but was unable.

I thought she needed to go out and helped her get to her feet.

But instead of going out, she just re-positioned herself in the dog bed and flopped down again.

"She's trying to get up," April commented, "and she can't."

My thoughts harkened back to that night I found Ini on my pile of clothes after the Sweat Lodge ceremony.

What about a little piece of joy for me? Why not? Didn't I deserve a little joy in life? There she was waiting for me. She didn't belong to anybody else.

For 12 years she had been nothing but pure joy... gift... blessing. As well as teacher.

It's impossible for me to willingly want you to go... in any other way than for God to take you.

But I don't want to see you have terrific pain - No.

I never want you to be away. Not one day, moment, second sooner.

But I am an adult. You are not getting better. You have this condition and you are only going to get worse. Why not save you from something terrible happening? It's the same end.

I agreed to the euthanasia appointment, and April scheduled it for 1 PM the following day...

CHAPTER FORTY-EIGHT

One with Ini...

The vain attempt to help her up had created a small amount of space for me to attempt to insert myself behind her and perhaps hold her.

I did that and it gave her ease.

I recalled the night before I took her to the emergency department, on that night in which she was urinating hour on the hour and looking so terrified, and she got in my bed, and I put my arms around her and held her, and she relaxed and slept through the night until I took her to the emergency room, and then got the cancer diagnosis.

Drifting into sleep, I had a dream, in which I saw Ini running in the park interacting with a lot of other dogs.

Then, waking up, I surveyed the room, looking for Ini; to my surprise, I saw several feet away by the side of the bed.

I wonder how she got there? I thought.

Then, as I went to get up, I found that I was still holding Ini with both my hands as she lay next to me.

What I'd seen by the bed was actually the crumpled brown sleeping bag I'd left to be with her.

And as for the real Ini, it was as though I was so used to holding her that she'd become a part of me...

CHAPTER FORTY-NINE

An exploration of grief...

Earlier in the day, I'd recalled that Blackie wasn't the first dog that had been taken away from me. There'd been a litter of puppies, and I'd got really attached to one that I called, "Cow", that had the same general color and disposition as Ini; and, in the end, my mother insisted, I let go of Cow, too.

April mistakenly thought that the puppies came from Blackie. That wasn't the case: First of all, Blackie was male. Second, the litter came from Joe's dog, Rover (And, no, I didn't think Blackie was the father; rather, Rover came to us pregnant).

"Oh, you had two dogs?" she responded. "What happened to Rover? Was she like Blackie and had to be given up?"

No, it was just only Blackie who went to the pound after biting that dog that would come into our backyard.

Meanwhile, Rover stayed in the house until the end and lived many years after that terrible night with Blackie: Blackie we gave up when I was in fifth grade. Rover was still with us when I went off to college.

Oddly, I essentially have no memories of Rover. Again, Rover was regarded as my brother's dog.

"So, wait," April said. "Joe's dog got to live in the house and have puppies. And your dog [Blackie] had to be tied up in the yard?"

There was more to it: Rover was acquired when we were still on Allott Avenue, and she was in the backyard with Blackie there (I remember that because that's where she had her litter of puppies – in a den that she dog in the fence line – I remember her keeping Blackie away from them).

But, yes, when we went to the new house in Studio City, Rover was brought into the house, whereas Blackie was tied to the tree in the backyard.

"And Rover wasn't both your dogs?" she clarified. "It could only be Joe's dog?"

Joe found Rover and brought Rover home, so she was recognized as Joe's dog.

"And you brought Blackie home?" she asked.

No, my mother brought Blackie home from her friend, Joyce's house. I remember the moment I saw him: A sweet little black puppy in a paper grocery sack.

"So, why was Blackie your dog?" April asked.

I didn't know. Maybe I just resonated with Blackie.

My brother and I were not close. That's just a statement of fact. Even as we occupied the same room growing up for all of our childhoods, our paths simply did not cross.

Indeed, my brother once told me, "if we weren't brothers, we wouldn't know each other..."

"Well, if we had had any kids, I would have never made one of the dogs one of the kids," she said. "They would be family dogs.

"I would never have one animal that supposedly belonged to one child be indoors, and the other one that belong to the other child be outdoors. That's not fair.

"And they would both be family dogs, and there would have to be a really good reason why one of them would always be outside. And it would have to do with their behavior."

I think the reason Blackie was delegated to outside was because he was seen as being too big to be in the house.

"Big?" she asked.

Yes, Blackie was a little bit bigger than Ini, and Rover was a little bit smaller than Ini. Blackie was probably 60 pounds, and Rover was probably 40 pounds.

In the end, I explain ours as having been a dysfunctional home, with a mother who didn't seem to know how to do a lot, and a husband who walked out on her/us, so she/we didn't have anyone to help her/us.

And my grandfather told my mother that she couldn't go home to be with family in New York because her kids were to acclimatized to the California climate and wouldn't be able to tolerate the harsh New York winters.

"Your mom wanted to go back to New York?"

I wasn't sure: It's hard to imagine that she wanted to be alone, but maybe she wanted her independence, too?

Or maybe it was because she was just stuck in inertia and wouldn't move… Literally.

I think of her as anxious and introverted and winding up alone.

And I took after my mother.

I turned to Ini.

"Ini, you look like Cow," I said. "You look like Cow. She was a sweet puppy. Just like you. It's like I got my Cow back. Precious girl."

"And I'm not a machine," April said, speaking for Ini. "I am not a machine, dad."

She was alluding to the toy dog that I bought with birthday money after Blackie was sent away to the pound.

"I'm not a toy dog, dad," April continued for Ini. "I'm real… "

CHAPTER FIFTY

Hamburger girl...

Outside, awaiting the hangman's arrival at the appointed hour, April recounted the story of Ini's first hamburger with friends.

"Mike was getting into skiing," she began, "and we were going with him, and we found this hotel that accepted dogs, and it was really, really nice. It was across the street from the Gondola, right in the center of town.

"So, Mike and his stepdaughter went up the gondola, and it was just me and Ini, and I'm walking around town looking at the restaurants, but there's Ini, so we can't go inside.

"But they have a bunch of restaurants where there's outdoor seating, and I found one where they had a fire going, and I found a table near the fire, and I ordered some food.

"And I saw on the menu a hamburger for dogs. So, I asked them, 'What does this mean?'

"And they said, 'Well, it's meat without any spices', and it was pretty inexpensive... I think it was three dollars? So, I thought, 'I'll get a hamburger for Ini.'

"And she ate it. And you could see that she went, 'Wow!'

"And then, every time we walked by that restaurant, she wanted to go in that restaurant. And I think months later, we did something similar, and she became a 'hamburger girl', because it gave her so much pleasure."

April commented that she'd been hearing about how people try to give their dog a great experience before they pass by serving them a steak or a hamburger.

"And we've been doing that for Ini for years," she said...

CHAPTER FIFTY-ONE

Ancestral, emotional support dog…

On the phone with our 'spirit buddy' (Steve), April talked about how it was that there was someone with Ini 24/seven, between herself, her mom and me.

"In addition, there have been a number of people who have come to visit ever since they found out that Ini has been on bedrest," she added. "And when they come to visit, she gets so excited that she can get up to pee."

April described how it was that Ini just want to be outside.

"So, we're spending all of our time outside on the front porch, with lots of coats and blankets and stuff," she began. "And I think love, a lot of care, Mike looking out for her, constantly cooking for her, a lot of social interaction, all those things all together have helped her rally.

"She's surrounded by love, she's surrounded by care, so that she gets right back. Like when she was experiencing this bloody diarrhea and she was really down and out physically, and Mike had to fight with the Emergency Room doctor to help her, and Mike came home really upset and he took to bed. And Ini got up on the bed, even though it was hard for her to do that. And she came as close as possible to him, and put her head over his knee, and she was just trying really hard to make him feel better.

"So, this is a dog who is in hospice, who is having bloody diarrhea, who is as miserable as can be – And she's doing everything she can to make Mike feel better, because he's emotionally upset. That's the kind of dog we're talking about."

"So, she earned all of this love," she concluded. "She earned it. She is just this ancestral, emotional support dog..."

CHAPTER FIFTY-TWO

Wonderful being...

"But the other thing that happened yesterday," April continued, "we had an appointment to euthanize Ini at 1 PM. But in the morning, she got up and she went to pee and she ate... She hadn't eaten the day before... And she was alert, so I was like, 'She's not ready to go.'

"So, we canceled the appointment, and different friends came, and one friend, Beth, came around five or six... We had a little belated Hanukkah celebration with her... It was lots of fun.

"But, then, Beth got in her car to drive home and something happened to her that she just accelerated her car and rammed it into another car... Yeah, so we hear the screech of tires going really fast and then the 'boom' of the car hitting the other car.

"So, we go down there to see what happened, and we see our friend's car wrapped around another car, and Ini runs to this car that's still going.

"So, I start screaming at Ini to stop, because the situation was kind of dangerous. And Ini wouldn't listen to me. Usually, she really listens to me when there's a panic in my voice. But she did not listen this time.

"So, I ran after her and I grabbed her, and I went to take her home. Because my mom was like, 'I'll take care of her', but Ini wouldn't leave.

"And the thing about it was, she ran faster than I've seen her run in a long time! This was a dog that wouldn't get out of bed by herself to go pee just like an hour or two before – And here she is jumping out of bed, running to the car, getting ready to help.

"She's just like this wonderful being..."

CHAPTER FIFTY-THREE

Shook out of fog?...

"And you know, Mike was amazing," April continued, expanding about the accident. "What happened was, something obviously went wrong in Beth's brain, because she basically got in her car and accelerated in the lane where you park and then slammed into the next car that was in front of her.

"But then when we went out there, she still had her foot on the gas. So, her car was still trying to run while it was impacted against this truck.

"So, there's smoke and there's a lot of friction going on there, and Mike opens the door to the driver side and helps Beth out of the car.

"So, Mike basically got a woman, a very confused woman, out of a smoking, moving vehicle. It was amazing."

"And Ini was right there trying to help her," Steve inserted. "And that got her up. That's wonderful."

"My mom has a theory," April commented. "That Ini got shook out of whatever fog or state she was in by the adrenaline of running to our neighbor..."

Postscript:

When the end came, Ini would again be shook out of her fog – And that would lead to perhaps the most difficult moment of my life...

CHAPTER FIFTY-FOUR

"Beautiful day..."

April continued telling Steve about Ini and the events of the day.

"She's wonderful," she said. "She's giving us this beautiful day in which she did all of the things that in the past few days I thought I'll never have again: She jumped in the bed with Cat Chow; She walked to the park; She chased squirrels; She did the evening walk and went to the corner and was protective of Cat Chow, waiting for her to catch up. Like all of the things that I just really treasure and I gave up on ever seeing again. They all happened in the past 24 hours..."

CHAPTER FIFTY-FIVE

Wave of grief...

"That is so beautiful!" Steve exclaimed. "She continues to give you these wonderful gifts. I mean, that was a gift today. It's almost as if she's doing it for you. She saying, 'Here, I know how much you love me. I want you to know how much I love you, too.'"

"Yeah, I was very calm and put a lot of effort to be in the moment and not being in the future and not looking at the future," April said. "Just being in the moment."

"I had a breakdown in the afternoon," she added, "because I suddenly let my mind go to the future and experienced this immense wave of grief, and I had to walk away.

"Now I have this taste of what my fate will be when she passes. And it's scary, because that was an immense wave of grief."

"But I got myself out of it," she concluded, "and had this great day today..."

CHAPTER FIFTY-SIX

Gift of knowing...

"Another gift Ini gave us over the last 24 hours," April continued, "is the gift of play. She brought out her toy and wants to play keep away and tug-of-war, even though she doesn't have a lot of oomph. I play with her like I play with a baby – Because I could obviously overpower her, but it's so much fun and brings up so much joy."

"It brings up joy for you and for her," Steve responded. "These are wonderful gifts. Wonderful, wonderful gifts."

"Yeah, and I think we're giving them to her," April commented. "We're giving her so much love and care that we're facilitating her reliving some of her most fun, cherished things that she loves about life."

"And it's the gift of knowing about what's going on with her," April concluded. "That Mike wound up taking her to UC Davis and found out the fate in store for us in time to have this period of sharing love..."

CHAPTER FIFTY-SEVEN

Euthanasia & non-human status?...

April talked about the issue of euthanasia.

"All of her doctors were pushing us really hard to euthanize," April said. "And to do it as soon as possible, and suggested the vets who come to your home, and to do it in the comfort of your home, rather than at the clinic, and presented going to the clinic is a lot more stressful.

"But the problem with these at home euthanasia people is that you have to schedule it in advanced and that they don't have spaces for same-day appointments. So, you basically have to call them and schedule in advance... For which I did, but then I canceled.

"But I don't think I'm going to do that again, because even though they say that if we do that, we save Ini from suffering... Well, I was thinking that Ini has the same status as a human, and we don't do that for humans... We don't schedule a human's death to save them from the suffering of death.

"I mean, if a human decided that that's what they wanted for themselves, then I would respect that and work with them on that. But if I don't know that that's what they want, I would never schedule their death.

"So, I decided I'm not doing that. When the end comes and she is suffering, we are five minutes away from a veterinarian hospital and we will try to get her there as soon as possible and get it done.

"But I am not going to schedule... I can't do it. It doesn't feel right. If she told me that's what she wanted, then I would honor it. But she can't tell me that she wants it. So, I'm just not doing it. I just can't. I hope I don't regret it... I tried it and it just doesn't feel right to me..."

CHAPTER FIFTY-EIGHT

She will let you know?...

"I think this is something that Ini will let you know when it is time," Steve responded. "She will let you know."

"And now, she is not there," he asserted. "She will let you know if she is in so much suffering that she cannot stand it. It's not time now. Absolutely not. And I think what you have planned is the smartest thing to do. She will let you know when she wants it..."

CHAPTER FIFTY-NINE

The rabbit card...

April shared her concern that there was another 'layer' in my experiences from my childhood that might make euthanasia difficult for me: When I was maybe seven years old, I had a rabbit; and some older neighborhood children came over and decided it would be good fun to slide the rabbit down our playset slide in the backyard. Initially, the rabbit resisted; but after a while, it stopped resisting; and after my "friends" left, the rabbit still wasn't moving; and when we took the rabbit to the vet, we were told that the rabbit was so scared by what happened to it, that it was not going to move again and had to be euthanized. It had literally been scared to death.

And that was the first and only animal that I saw euthanized. And to this day I remember what I saw... It was like the light in the animal was snuffed out.

Naturally, the reason that April is so concerned is because this was not a pleasant experience, and now we were looking at the euthanasia of my favorite spiritual being - This doggie who has only given me unconditional love and who I love in return, and what that was bringing up in me at an emotional level?

I have been telling April that it really isn't that complex, and we don't have to worry about any "layers" from traumatic experiences in my childhood.

But maybe I was mistaken?

"It makes me think of the medicine cards," Steve commented, "which are animals - like a nature deck. And rabbit is the 'fear card.' And for a long time, I thought, 'Oh, I don't want to get rabbit in my reading.' Because that's like calling up your fears."

"And then one day, it dawned on me that fear is never called up until it's ready to be healed," he concluded. "So, when the fear is called up, it's ready to be healed…"

CHAPTER SIXTY

"Priority on the helper..."

As I previously indicated, my mother-in-law, Doris, was being intensely helpful to us during this process, and a steadying force where April and I were concerned.

Earlier, I alluded to April making the statement about her mother having a theory about how Ini was able to transition from a non-ambulatory to running at the time of our neighbor's accident. Now, I'm going to offer my mother-in-law's words to elaborate:

"When your neighbor got in trouble and crashed that car into the truck, Ini was able to connect with her own need to be helpful, even as she was in so need of help. She had received help and accepted help from your neighbor in the food she brought over. So, there was this connection. And then, Ini just rose to the occasion when your neighbor needed help."

"I think it definitely gave her something," my mother-in-law continued. "Again, I go back to the example of my father: My father had been a psychoanalyst [Indeed, he trained under Sigmund and Anna Freud]... Well, later in life, he had a stroke; and while he was in the hospital, whether it was his stroke or depression, we thought we had lost him.

"And then this patient came and said, 'I need you, doctor'; and dad sent my mother and me away; and an hour later, when we came back, he was back! He was back to being the helper... He was also the helped, but priority on the helper - To be needed..."

Postscript:

In my work with homeless veterans, I'd always contended that just as important as shelter and medical assistance is the need to be of service. That's why I've always supported the Compensated Work Therapy program, which gives these veterans the opportunity to perform meaningful work...

CHAPTER SIXTY-ONE

Heart-to-heart...

Performing Bioenergy with Ini just now, there was an interesting movement of the energy – Going from her heart to my heart, and back to her heart.

At present, she is not eating or drinking. She has not since one in the morning. And I don't know why? I especially don't know why she's not drinking?

What would make someone stop that? I think to myself. Stomach? Throat? Is she suffering? No doubt she's suffering. What to do? Would she please just slip away?

Meanwhile, I'm angry at April, because a short time ago, just as I got Ini up in the harness [She'd been struggling every other minute to get up!] and it seemed like she would pee, April good-naturedly called to her and interrupted the process.

"Hi, Ini, how are you?" she said in her usual cheerful way.

After that, Ini insisted on walking back to her dog bed without having relieved herself.

But I wouldn't allow myself to openly voice my disappointment, because it would upset Ini, and now she doesn't have the strength to run away from my negative energy.

And I'm staying with her in the place that make her feel happy... In the front of the house, with the sun and nature and brightly colored yellow leaves falling from our magnificent mulberry tree.

Ini is looking out good-naturedly, as though to offer a message that says, "There is always a way and a reason to be joyful", and I can honor Ini by being that way.

And at that very thought, lo and behold, my chest becomes all puffed out and expanded (where it's usually sunken) and air filling my lungs, such that I believe it couldn't have happened any other way than through connecting with Ini's energy and that message.

I want to be joyful and happy.

Ini has shown me the way...

CHAPTER SIXTY-TWO

"...she's seen you get to a good point in your life..."

"Ini is in suffering mode," my wise friend, Sam, began, "and resting and doing that final rest may be the best thing. Because what you may see may not be the full picture. And you just have to make sure your eyes are open when you do make that decision, because maybe Ini's ready?"

He had called to check on me. I wouldn't know how prophetic his words were until my last hour with Ini.

"That's a tough place that you're in right now," he continued. "But it's just a matter of time now.

"But I think you're sure lucky to have Ini. I mean, isn't it incredible?... She came into your life at the right time, and she's seen you get to a good point in your life."

That she had.

The following came from my first book about Ini, in which I shared with a Native American woman what happened that drove me to the Indian Reservations where Ini chose me:

"I ran afoul with the clinic where I was working – a place called FQHC. I accepted the job there because April's grandmother was dying, and the clinic was nearby. The grandmother was all but mother to April; this way she could be there for her grandmother's final days.

"I was an experienced physician. Before FQHC I'd been a medical director with the Tennessee Health Department; I'd received commendations from Health Department for transforming the worst community medical center in the state to a model of excellence.

Given those past achievements, I couldn't imagine having a problem at FQHC.

"But I guess you could say I didn't understand the ground rules. FQHC stands for Federally Qualified Health Center. They receive most of their funding from the government. I thought at a place like this, standard of care would be the norm. But the doctors there were doing a lot of questionable things. Tons of money wasted on unnecessary tests, referrals, and imaging studies. Worst of all was all the narcotic prescribing. Vicodin, Darvon, Percocet being doled out like candy. When I'd be asked to cover for these other doctors, I'd perform urine drug screens to determine if their patients were taking these medications appropriately. Inevitably, results showed that the narcotics weren't in their system – What was showing up was heroin and cocaine. And here FQHC was right next to a school. Instead of part of the solution, it felt like FQHC was part of the problem, and rather than working to keep national healthcare afloat, it was sinking it."

"I was having nightmares," I continued. "In one of them, I was at a waterpark with my colleagues; they were sliding their children down waterslides. But instead of water, the slides were streaming blood, and all of them were covered in it. Looking at them, they were smiling; seemingly having a good time with their wives and children. I stood pleading, 'Guys, this isn't right.'

"I awoke from that dream knowing I had to do something and went right to my Clinical Director and insisted he act to correct those problems...

"Not long after I went to the Clinical Director, though, I became the target for every kind of inquiry and investigation. They told me all my cases were being reviewed and if a hundred percent didn't meet their satisfaction, I'd be terminated. Over the ensuing weeks, they really made an example out of me. They moved me from cubicle to cubicle. Put me in rooms right next to construction; sledgehammers operating essentially right next to me. Finally, they placed me on a forced leave of absence while they 'considered' my position. A week later I received my termination notice."

"How could they do that?" she asked. "When you were doing your job?"

"They could do what they wanted," I responded, matter-of-factly. "Even though it was a federally-qualified health center subsidized by the government, it was privately owned. I'd signed an 'at-will' contract in a 'right-to-work' state. I had no recourse..."

So, Sam was right: From the lowest point in my life when I'd been reduced to fighting for my career, to now when I was about to realize my dream of working to attempt to validate my calling in life (i.e., Bioenergy and Chi Gong) at an Ivy League institution, Ini had been there.

"You know, really, there are a lot of struggles that you have to go through," Sam continued. "But, overall, you're so much further ahead then you've ever been in your life. And Ini has been a part of that - Which is remarkable."

Yes, Ini had even showed me the way when it came to the promise that Bioenergy and Chi Gong held.

The following comes from the latest version of my Bioenergy Handbook, in which I documented Ini's role in showing me what Medical Chi Healing was capable of in the way of massive resets and muscular releases.

...Ini developed a condition called Granulocytic Meningomyeloencephalitis (GME), a condition whereby the immune system attacks the nerves throughout the body, resulting in generalized pain, fever, incoordination, seizures and depression for weeks, with most dogs not surviving it.

Fortunately, we found a veterinarian who specialized in Neurology and Neurosurgery, who pulled Ini through; however, even after her condition was stabilized with immunosuppressants, Ini was still racked with pain. Her nerve endings had been effectively fried everywhere. Indeed, people who suffer from something equivalent to her condition (like arachnoiditis) usually require massive doses of steroid and narcotic medication to tolerate the associated pain.

Then, later, when Ini was referred to an Integrative Medicine specialist who learned about my expertise in Chi Gong, he suggested I perform Medical Chi Healing on Ini.

For weeks I did this on a daily basis and saw no change in Ini's condition. Then, one day, after performing Medical Chi Healing, Ini's whole body looked to be doing the equivalent of 'the wave.' It wasn't anything like the typical twitches and fasciculations that accompany a dog's sleep; rather, her whole body was moving like a sine wave – VOOM! VOOM! VOOM! – over and over again. It was as though some switch had been flipped and the result was this massive reset that involved every muscle in her body – contracting and relaxing in one major wave after another.

And when the process was through, she was a different dog: she could tolerate being petted, which she hadn't before because the nerves have been so sensitized; she could tolerate heat or sunlight, which she hadn't since the start of the condition; and she was relatively free of pain!

"She not only came back from the dead," a colleague commented. "She turned into a pup. Your slow process of addressing one problem at a time, doing Medical Chi Healing every day, led to that massive reset. Because then all of a sudden everything just snaps together. It's like spontaneous combustion. It's like how we evolved. There was this primordial soup and then the molecules just came together. But it took years and years. It was a slow process. But then once it matched up, then it was just like an explosion – BOOM! – and then things quickly accelerate and suddenly start happening.

"I think that's the way our body works, too. We just slowly ascend so we don't over pressurize from a dive, but then when we reach the surface, we breakthrough..."

"She's been in that phase of yours of growth and finding yourself and hoping that you become a better person," Sam continued. "So, my gosh, she probably feels like, 'Yep, I did my job. I did it well.'

Did she ever.

The thing is, though – In her final moments and after, she would wind up teaching me even more lessons and contribute to my growth in ways I'm still trying to process...

"Ini has made me think of all the dogs I had," Sam continued. "They've all been very special throughout my life. And with you at this crossroads here, it just reminds me of the crossroads I've been at, and how wonderful their influences have been with me. And I feel very fortunate, and very, very lucky to have known them all. And to have had them really make a mark on me in a very, very positive way. I'm very fortunate."

"I know you're probably on a very thin thread holding you up," he concluded. "But it's a strong spider thread, so it will hold you..."

CHAPTER SIXTY-THREE

When she's relaxed...

Ini has made her wishes clear: What she wants is to be with us.

April walked away, and I went and followed her to discuss Ini's fate? And returning, Ini was wide awake and waiting for us, with Ima saying Ini did not relax until she saw us again.

"That's when she relaxed," Doris said.

What she wants is to be with us. That's what gives her ease...

Probably more than some stranger injecting her with some euthanasia cocktail. And that doesn't seem such a difficult request to fulfill for a being who has been as loving to us as Ini has.

And at the same time as she was getting what she wanted, she was giving me exactly what I wanted: Her company. Her presence.

Just like she did in every long car ride, when I got to enjoy her presence and her scent.

And it probably didn't matter what I did; she just wanted my company. Even now that she wasn't able to enjoy treats while sitting next to my desk, or squirrels while sitting next to me at the park. She just wants my company.

And I want her company.

"We'll get through this, Ini," I said...

CHAPTER SIXTY-FOUR

Lymphadenopathy

Ini is developing some significantly enlarged lymph nodes along places in her body, like her neck and axilla.

It can't be comfortable, I thought. With lymph nodes like these, it must be like having the flu.

Only probably a hell of a lot worse. It's probably among the reasons she's so anxious and uncomfortable during the night...

CHAPTER SIXTY-FIVE

"Low energy day"
Wednesday, December 20, 2023

April talked about Ini having had a "low energy day", in which she spent most of the day sleeping.

I don't mind: Ini is, as April would say, "scouting out the next world in her dreams."

And it's a world that I want her to go to!

So, she could spend as much time there as she wants as far as I'm concerned.

Just as long as she's not suffering...

CHAPTER SIXTY-SIX

"You can let go"

As I'm making my way through this time, I'm having these really intense spontaneous releases at my solar plexus ("the seat of emotions").

I feel I'm connecting with Ini.

And the message seems to be, "Letting go is OK. This spirit entity is still in your heart. You can let her go to whatever world they're going to. It's OK..."

CHAPTER SIXTY-SEVEN

Imprinted connection...

Doris commented that just watching me stroke Ini's fur, she had a visceral feeling for the deep love and care I felt for Ini.

"I had a little bit of that, as well," she said, "where I was able to stop her fidgeting. But not like you can. I definitely see your connection."

"I mean, you're like her birth mother," she added. "I should probably say father.... But you were imprinted on her... From puppyhood.

"And you also have a spiritual understanding, too. So, this energetic connection you have with her just speaks to me.... And I think it speaks to her, too."

"Sometimes we need to let go of the things we care about," she concluded. "It's a lesson I never learned..."

CHAPTER SIXTY-EIGHT

"Most amazing, best Reservation dog ever..."

"Do you remember when she used to be your dog?" April asked. "And then you got so into the Headquarters job that she became my dog.

"And then she became our dog. Do you remember?"

I was so busy back then that I didn't even know what they did during the day while I was at Headquarters?

"I think I spent a lot of time looking for housing, which was pretty much impossible, because it was so moldy and all those places," April said. "And we spent a lot of time together. We'd go to the park. We'd go to the dog park.

"I would go to the art studio sometimes... but I wasn't that active there... because I just wanted to be with Ini... I didn't want to separate. I just wanted to be with her. I'd rather do that than do my art.

"I suppose I could have had a home studio and done my art,... But not really... An art studio is no place for a dog – with all those toxic fumes."

I thought about all the fun that April and Ini had been. What a good life they had made for me.

"You get an A+ plus, plus, plus," April commented of Ini. "You're the most amazing, best Reservation dog ever..."

CHAPTER SIXTY-NINE

Dirge...

"Thank you for always wanting to go anytime we were going somewhere," April told Ini.

Just being with her was like being with a little package of joy everywhere, I added.

"I'm so sorry you had all of these illnesses," April continued. "And I'm so sorry I was kind of rough as a nurse. It all came out of love and wanting to have you and to make you well and maintain as much of your health as possible.

"We didn't understand why these illnesses were doing all of these things, but we were just trying to help.

"I'm sorry for the times I was sticking things in your mouth and cleaning up places that hurt.

"And I'm sorry I couldn't explain to you why I was doing these things to you. I hope you're not angry."

Of course, she wasn't angry at April, I thought.

"Sorry we didn't catch this with some time to be able to have a way to fix this," she continued. "I'm sorry that you've spent two months suffering without us knowing what was going on.

"We did take you to the doctor's... And it was a really good doctor... We took you to several doctors during those two months... But, I don't know?... I guess we didn't tell them the right things?..."

CHAPTER SEVENTY

Difficulty breathing.
Thursday, December 21, 2023

Ini wouldn't drink today. I didn't know why? This was certainly something that Ini never manifested before – Indeed, it was the antithesis of everything she'd manifested.

But it was true. Something (whether it was localized at her throat and related to the neurologic messages from her brain) was keeping her from drinking.

As such, I felt it was only a matter of time before she slipped away.

However, though her weakness had progressed, she was repeatedly indicating she wanted to get up. As such, using the harnesses, I lifted her over and over, and directed her like a marionette to the lawn in vain efforts to help her relieve herself.

Though, even in this, Ini provided joy and healing, because although it wasn't easy to manipulate her in that harness to the lawn to do her business, instead of injury coming from all of that, healing did, as my back muscles just became activated and then released.

Hence, what I thought would provoke harm and injury, wound up providing healing, as my body loves to be used, and what had turned it into a dysfunctional mess was actually the academic pattern that I'd been pushed into by those who did not know how to attend my childhood injuries...

Meanwhile, after a full day without eating or drinking, Ini finally had some water just before it was time for all of us to go to bed.

As usual, Ini had preferred to spend the day outside on the front patio, so April and I put out some sleeping bags, intent on spending the night outdoors with her.

Then, at one in the morning, a thick fog came rolling in, and April felt the dampness wasn't good for Ini and insisted we all go inside.

That's when she gave me the news.

"I think Ini's having difficulty breathing," she said.

Indeed, her breathing was labored and she was making use of her abdominal muscles.

This was a redline: We weren't going to let Ini suffer air hunger and suffocation.

We lifted her into the car and took her to the pet hospital...

CHAPTER SEVENTY-ONE

"Whack..."

At the pet hospital, the veterinarian on-call only had to look at Ini to know what was needed.

Nevertheless, he thoughtfully asked what we wanted?

I said I wanted to know the cause of Ini's turn for the worse.

The vet was kind, and instead of performing a million-dollar workup, he started by performing a relatively simple procedure called an arterial blood gas (ABG), which provides about the most accurate information about the body's state of oxygenation, as well as the internal machinations for that.

The results of the ABG, though, were jaw dropping, as the acid-base disturbances suggested an inordinate amount of multi-organ failure with metabolic disorders of her system that ran the gamut of everything from respiratory failure to diabetic complications to cancer complications and everything in between!

"So, what you're saying is," April interjected. "All of the systems in her are going whack..."

CHAPTER SEVENTY-TWO

"Something right..."

"It was game over," April would later say of that ABG. "Mike didn't even know how to approach it. He was like, 'I have no idea what's going on. I've never heard or seen readings like this before...'"

In my forty years of medical training and patient experience, I had never encountered an ABG as complex and complicated as this. At the very least, it explained Ini's alternating pattern of deep sleep to complete wakefulness, as a manifestation of electrical brain wave shifts caused by these metabolic disturbances.

"That sounds like she's really suffering," April commented.

Yes, she was. There was a reason she was looking at me so anxiously in the night.

But she just worked so hard at being with us until the end. It was just a mark of how much she loved us and wanted to be with us.

"I must have done something right as her mama," April said...

CHAPTER SEVENTY-THREE

No other option...

Even on supplemental oxygen, Ini wasn't achieving oxygenation levels compatible with life. As such, the only options were relieve her suffering by euthanasia, or hospitalize her – Though the latter would only stabilize her condition and she couldn't come home with us again. As such, there was really no other option than euthanasia.

Waiting for the vet to bring Ini into the room with us to perform the procedure, April and I reflected on what a gift Ini had been to us.

"We had her for 12 years," April said.

Yes, great years, in which every moment was a source of joy.

"I mean, I picked her over my art over and over again," April continued. "I'd rather just be with her."

Any time I had wanted to go out into the "wild places", the first person I wanted to turn to was Ini. It was she I was so used to going with me into the wild places: The lovely places to look out at; to enjoy and appreciate; to travel with a friend and companion, who enjoys nature as much as I do; the sights and sounds. It was all just great and impossible to be better.

She was my beloved girl; pretty as a picture. How lucky I have been... To have had that beautiful girl with me all of these years...

And she loved me, too. I was her dad. When another dog came around, it was, "Uh, uh, no. This is my dad."

How lucky I had been.

And she was kind enough to be with me all the time that I wasn't at work, whether it was a walk into the fields in the Northern Plains or sitting at my side while I wrote my books.

And every car ride, in which I could enjoy her scent and having her there…

Then, they wheeled Ini in on a gurney and offered to give us some time before the euthanasia procedure.

She was calm at first, but then I was struck by how alert Ini looked when they wheeled her back to us.

It was not unlike what happened that night our neighbor crashed her car into the back of that truck, and Ini somehow "sprung into action" and from, as April would say, "fleeting away" to being fully back in her body again.

"Yeah, because she was kind of sullen on the trip over here," April said. "And she was lying down when they brought her into the room again. But when she saw us, it was like she woke up.

"And I'm wondering if it isn't because she walked into a room that smelled of distress; and she saw that all three of us were distressed and it was just her instinct to come to you when you were distressed?"

Indeed, I wasn't happy about April's weeping. I felt it was a time to be strong for Ini, and reassuring about sending her pleasantly onwards to her next journey, and not infecting her with any sadness.

In any event, it had the effect of activating Ini again, so that we had her fully "back."

And so the stage was set for what would be perhaps the most difficult and heart-wrenching experience I would ever have…

Postscript:

In retrospect, though, as stated, it was all terribly heart-wrenching, it's also what made Ini a saint. It was her final test in selflessness and rising to display a capacity for love rivaled by none…

CHAPTER SEVENTY-FOUR

Compassion from a stranger...

"She doesn't want to go," April said. "She's begging to be let off the gurney. She's begging us to let her stay with us. She's wanting to stay with us, even though she's suffering..."

I asked the emergency room doctor to please give us some time?

He kindly submitted to our request. Indeed, he had been so very good to us, treating us compassionately, willing to evaluate it step-by-step, so that we could come to terms with what had to be.

And here he was someone who we hadn't met before, working the night shift from midnight to six in the morning, willing to help these total strangers through such a painful, heart-wrenching process.

"He knew what was best for her," April said...

"I think it's because we're so upset," April commented. "She was feeling like crap, but then her people were so upset.

"And that's the way she is. Whenever we're upset, she runs to us.

"The reason she wants to get up is to come to us.

"She isn't looking at the door. She's looking at us. She's reacting to the fact that we were upset."

Yes, she cares about us...

"I was reading up about dogs," April continued. "That they could smell your distress. Like you emit chemical signals when you're upset and dogs have the capability of smelling your distress.

"And we had been sitting in that room for a while before she was wheeled back here. We have been in here for hours - when the doctor came in and talk to us, and then when he told us about the test, and then we made the decision to..."

She choked up.

"So, she got wheeled in, and she probably got slammed with that smell of us being so upset.

"And it woke her up. It got her out of whatever state she was in. And she's like, 'You're so upset. How can I help?'

"She rallied because we're so upset...."

CHAPTER SEVENTY-FIVE

A view of Ini's last moments...

April described Ini's last moments.

"She looked at you so intently," she said. "I was trying to look at her face, but I didn't see her eyes - She was so focused on you."

Yes, I saw it all.

And I felt my crown chakra pop just before she received the injection.

Still, I wasn't expecting what happened in between...

CHAPTER SEVENTY-SIX

Parting message...

April inquired what unexpected happening occurred at the moment of the injection?

I had been looking in Ini's eyes, and the message she imparted was, "Dad, I never want to leave you. Dad, I always wanted to stay with you."

Then, she looked up to God, and that was it.

That gets to be my parting memory from my beloved doggie:

"Dad, I never want to leave you. Dad, I always want to stay with you..."

CHAPTER SEVENTY-SEVEN

"...wasn't going to go out quietly..."

"I always want to be with you, too," April commented, tearfully. "I have worked for five years to avoid this moment."

She asked if this was different from my experience with the bunny?

Yes, with the bunny, it's life just went out like turning off a light switch.

But not Ini: She would not be turned out like a lightbulb; she would insist on illuminating the whole universe before she went out.

"She wasn't going to go out quietly," April agreed.

Then, she broke down and cried.

"But there was nowhere else to take her," she concluded. "Because things were closing in on her at all sides, and they were not compatible with life..."

CHAPTER SEVENTY-EIGHT

Deserving of reverence...

I commented that, in her last moments, Ini not only taught me how to live, she taught me how to die.

"What do you mean?" April asked. "Because she's so strong?"

Yes. Dying is never easy. None of us knows what comes after this life. She wanted to stay. And I'm probably gonna want to stay to the last second, too.

Here I am, someone who knows what it is to nearly die - Someone who knows in his heart what the next life involves.

And yet, I cling to life.

But there is a time to go. There is a time to let go of suffering.

And maybe I could be like Ini, and when I go, share a lot of love - Like Ini constantly imparted to me in this process. She just wanted to give love the whole time.

That's what she showed me: That you could live a life of just giving love to the last.

That deserves my reverence...

CHAPTER SEVENTY-NINE

"Loving in spite of us?..."

I shared my veterinarian-friend's comment about pets ("I think they live for us").

But April disagreed.

"I don't think all dogs are like that," she said. "She... She... It didn't matter what we did to her. What I did to her."

She looked at me.

"How many people want to love the person sticking stuff down your throat every day?" she asked. "I did things every day that were not pleasant to her. I..."

April broke off, then offered some retrospective thoughts.

"I wish they hadn't left us in that exam room," she said, "and put us in this room that's particularly for euthanasia.

"Or that I would have had the presence of mind to just put her on the dog bed, with us just sitting around her."

Yes, given her some morphine, to treat the air hunger and let her slowly fade away.

Just like your treat a human person in their last moments.

But that isn't what veterinarians do. They euthanize animals. And, so, you just kill the animal.

In the end, it permitted Ini to earn her wings 100 times over. As this amazing being who is just so capable of love, so to always be awakened by the call to help those she loved.

To be willing to endure the worst suffering to abide and rise to the call to help those she loved.

All the way to the last minute.

April hesitated, then suggested that we sing some Lakota prayer songs...

CHAPTER EIGHTY

Chorus of doubt...

Not unlike the time that Ini and I got caught in the white-out, I found myself feeling crazed with competing thoughts as I stepped outside the pet hospital.

You and me, Ini, I thought. Going out into the wilds of the Northern Plains, no matter whether it was a summer day or a winter blizzard, and having a wonderful time. All alone facing the elements. Alone but together. All the sights and sounds to take in. I always wanted you with me. Why didn't I always keep you with me?

I say to myself, "It's because you had to die. You just had to. It was the cancer. It was only a matter of time before it was going to get you. And it was going to keep eating away at you. It was going to keep on getting worse for you. Wasting you away and reducing you to nothing."

Now you can always be beautiful in my eyes.

But who cares? Who in the world would care what you look like? How could it be that I care about such a triviality? How could I be that superficial? Especially when really, the memory I'm always going to have is of you looking to God and seemingly saying to me, "Daddy, I love you. Daddy, I always want to be with you. Daddy, I never want to leave you." That will be my enduring memory. Not the sleepy dog for whom you just turn off the lights and deliver the death medicine. No. It didn't happen that way. It was my dog all full of life, telling me that she still wanted to live.

Yes, I didn't want you in pain. Yes, I didn't want to see you stumble and get hurt. I didn't.

But did I do that more for me than for you? Maybe so.

Can you forgive me? Of course, you can. And of course, you will. That's just your nature. Love.

But what of me? How will I live with myself? With looking in your eyes, begging for more time with me, and me not insisting on that for you and me? Just providing a cold goodbye and it's time to move on? Because it's too hard and I don't want to watch it anymore?

I think of my co-worker, Manny, who told me the story about his dog getting sick and his taking it to the vet:

"The vet said, 'I can help your dog, but it will cost $3000," Manny began. "I said, 'I ain't got no $3000 for a dog. How much would it cost to put the dog down?... $60... Put the dog down...'"

And Manny had a generous heart - He gave money to the poor any time he saw them. He had a heart for the homeless. He was as humanitarian a person as they get. He/we just live in the world. We're stuck here living in the world. And for the common men, there are choices in life. There are the things you do; the things you have to do; and everything else. You do the best you can...

Those who are strong enough to want to embrace life for all it's worth, in spite of the pain, find a way to do so up until that last moment.

Ini did.

Ini, if you're willing, hold onto that love, and I'll try to be even more loving in the next life.

I will reach out to you in the void, or maybe it won't be as tough as you think; and we'll all be in a place of love soon, where we can laugh at all of these travails; And then maybe we can embrace them again, and dare to live in the physical plane once more, with all its suffering and hardship, and fight for survival, so to have an opportunity to better learn the lessons of the universe, like we couldn't sitting on that cloud and reading about it in the spirit world. Ini, throughout our years together, you have taught me lessons; But this lesson... This is the hardest of all.

I kept praying and begging God that you would just slip away. And then when you developed that labored breathing, I knew that euthanasia was what had to be done. There was no question. All of the medical advice, all of the medical evaluations - They all pointed to that.

But, then, when it happened, what occurred? – "Daddy, I love you. Daddy, I always want to be with you. Daddy, I never want to leave you." I was not expecting that. I was just wanting her to have relief... And feel some joy in that relief.

But, no. She loved her life so much with us that even with all that pain and agony, she wanted to stay.

There was no, "Oh, thank God, you finally decided to let me go." Not for Ini.

They say for the great ones that death has to be hard, because it has to be one more final trial for them to face and rise to and overcome.

So, Ini earned her place, as one of the great ones.

But did you have to be so incredible and want to be with us even in all of that suffering?

She was too good for this world. She was really too good for this world. Because there is not enough sanctity for life in this world to honor a spirit like her.

She should have been honored at every moment. People should have been bowing down praying to keep her alive. Here was this being who was so capable of being willing to suffer to give love. even I wasn't willing to bow down in respect of that.

It was though Ini were saying, "Dad, I would have given you the world - Given you health; Given you love; Someone who loves you more than anyone - Who never wanted to leave you. I would have given you all that in spades. Wouldn't that have been worth the thousands of dollars in hospitalization costs, if even for only a few days? What's money anyways? Yeah, the doctors told you, 'It doesn't make any sense', but what is the value of love to you? Wouldn't that have been something worth paying for? Isn't every moment of that worth paying for?" How would I live with myself when my last memory of Ini alive was that look in her eye, seemingly beseeching God for assistance and indicating she wanted to stay with us?...

It's as though all I am is still my father's son, for whom the apple has not fallen far from the tree. And when it requires too much effort or investment, or when it's too inconvenient, I just put you down...

The pain associated with that night made me understand how it was that people could do stupid things. Get fat on "comfort food." Because they need comfort.

They take drugs. They have sex. Get themselves into all kinds of trouble. Because they need comfort from all the things that of happened to them. And how hard life was to them. From how brutally hard life is.

They probably all know better, but they can't do better. They get themselves into patterns because it seems to provide some temporary relief and it even might be a little bit fun at times.

Otherwise, they don't have the skills to be able to recover from these terrible things that they've seen and experienced.

And I am going to go out there and try to give them a skill for that. With something that I am especially capable of teaching and

training them to do...

CHAPTER EIGHTY-ONE

Words of solace...

April noticed that I was distressed and asked what was the matter?

I said those last moments with Ini were haunting me, such that I felt I'd missed the mark.

"By not keeping her alive?" she asked. "No, no, no, no, no, no. No. She couldn't breathe. She couldn't breathe. And they didn't know why? And they didn't think the x-rays were going to tell us. They didn't even want to do x-rays on her. They didn't want to have to analyze her. They would have done it if you told them to, but they didn't want to. Because she couldn't breathe and it could be all sorts of different, bizarre things.

"There were too many holes in the dam. She didn't have the strength. She couldn't walk anymore. And she didn't want any medical stuff... We would have brought her home and watched her choke to death."

"What you saw could have been a reaction to stress," April asserted. "Because she's been on gurneys before and it meant surgery and things like that? And maybe it was just stress from being at the hospital? So, maybe it was more like she was saying, 'Take me home, because I don't want to be in this hospital', instead of, 'I want to stay. I want to stay here suffering, and then have even more suffering.'

"I just had an inner feeling of, 'It's time. She's just suffering. Let's do it as soon as possible.'

"When the doctor came and you were like, 'Metabolically, it makes no sense. They're not supportive of life. It's just multiple system failure – like all of her systems are failing', then that really got inside of me, so I felt like, 'It's time to let go', and that feeling like we shouldn't wait got really strong.

"And, also, the Vet was looking at us in this way that you knew he thought that it was past time. So, he was giving us this feeling like it was past time.

"I just got that feeling inside of me of, 'She's suffering. It's time. Nothing is going to make it any better. And the longer I hold onto her, she's just going to suffer.'"

April broke down in tears...

CHAPTER EIGHTY-TWO

Order of things...

April talked about the order with which she, Ini and I used to walk along the trails.

"There was always Ini between us," she said. "She following you, and I'm following her, because I want to make sure she was OK."

I guess Ini was following me because she wanted to make sure I was OK, I commented.

April laughed.

I added I'd like to think it was because I was a halfway decent playmate.

"You were," April agreed. "You were. You were. You were. You were lots of fun."

"That's why she basically looked to you in the last moments," she concluded. "You took on that burden..."

CHAPTER EIGHTY-THREE

"She's getting in the car!..."

April pleated her hair into a braid to bury with Ini.

"It's going away, but when I was young, my hair had 'fire' in it," she said. "It had this copper fire to it. And Ini also has copper fire."

Then, she gave me a scissors and instructed me to cut her hair.

After doing so, she asked if I wanted her to cut some of my hair to bury with Ini?

I said I did.

On the question of burial procedure, April asked what I thought Ini would prefer?

"Merge with all of nature and other lifeforms and be a part of the lifecycle and all that?" she asked. "Or would she want to come with us in her inorganic form?"

The answer was unquestionably to be with us.

"She's getting in the car!" April said, mimicking what she'd say when Ini would always insist on going with us any time we were making plans to travel somewhere.

"She's getting in the car!" April repeated through her tears now...

CHAPTER EIGHTY-FOUR

Sending healing energy...

The veterinarian staff brought us to a room to spend more time quietly with Ini.

In the dimly lit and well-furnished room reserved for those who recently lost a pet, there was a bowl containing memorial lapel pins featuring the figure of a dog with angel wings.

Yes, she got her wings, I thought. In spite of her system shutting down and her not being able to breathe, the feeling I got from her in those last moment was, "I want to stay. I love you and I want to stay."

"Yeah," April said. "Yeah, she wanted to stay. She wanted to be with us. She wanted to get up and leave the hospital. She wanted to get off that gurney."

It took an outside force to take her out of our lives. It took medicine – or poison – or whatever you want to call it. Because her will was such that it could only be that way that she would part with us.

There have been those who told me that the great souls are tested and have to endure a hard death before they reach Nirvana... Well, that's how Ini left this world.

It was against her will, so that some other force has to snuff out that light. Because her light was so great that she was willing to endure anything... Any agony... To be with those she loved.

It was unforgettable. That she could love that much and show that much strength to want to endure that way.

Some people say there's no good death. But if you ask me, that was a good death.

"The thing about Ini's death was that she was surrounded with love," April said. "On a daily basis, all of her friends came by to visit her. Lee came. And Beth came. And Caroline came. And then a few other people came. And Dino came. And Kino came. So, she was just surrounded with love and care. So, when the time came, she knew that she was not alone."

And not only was she loved by everyone, she loved back.

I bent low and kissed Ini behind her ear, the way I always had before leaving her; however, now, I felt the cold there that had never been there before.

I scanned Ini energetically and felt her energy/Qi flowing into my crown chakra.

April indicated she was feeling something, too.

"You know how she wasn't interested in getting out of the car when you would drive her?" she began. "Well, this one time, I sat with her, and I was petting her outside in the garage. And I was doing this for a long time, and as I was petting her, I was thinking about how my heart was going to get ripped open. And she told me not to worry, because she was going to send me light, and it was going to fill up the part of my heart that got ripped."

"And that's what I was feeling just now," she asserted. "Like you were giving me that good energy and it was going to my heart, like she had told me that she was going to do."

Yes, I could feel that, going through me, through my crown chakra, to April.

"So, there is light filling in where the tear in my heart is," she concluded...

CHAPTER EIGHTY-FIVE

Taking Ini home…

We decided to take Ini home. We were told she would be placed in a casket, and we drove around to the delivery area, waiting for Ini to be brought out to us. A big trans fella brought the casket with Ini and placed it in the back of the car.

April was concerned about the way this fella was carrying the casket (pressed to his chest), wondering how it would affect Ini's body position? I, meanwhile, had previously observed this fella carrying dogs back-and-forth to treatment rooms, and I'd appreciated the full-body manner in which he would hold them (like hugging them) on their way to getting care. So, I didn't mind that his handling might have affected Ini's position in the casket; I was happy that he'd been holding her in his caring arms.

Indeed, his handling of her seemed not unlike the way that I had whisked Ini away from the sweat lodge grounds on that night she chose me, and she sank into my arms… Like she had a feeling she was going someplace good and didn't have to be afraid, even though she had no idea where this person was taking her.

"She wanted you," April commented. "She needed a person…"

CHAPTER EIGHTY-SIX

"Ini inspires…"

At the house, April, Doris and I decided to decorate the casket using colored markers and quotes about how 'Ini inspired.'

"Your memory inspires us to be joyful in play… be friendly to strangers… smile in adversity… to want to help and leave no one behind… to insist on really yummy food… to offer comfort freely… to spread love and joy… to be ready to go on an adventure… to look on others with soft eyes… to find a gentle way… to protect those who love and look after them… to visit friends daily..."

"And enjoy treats!" April added, spiritedly. "But I guess that's part of yummy food…"

CHAPTER EIGHTY-SEVEN

Ini's message...

    With Ini's passing, there's been something of a mantra playing in my head: "Enjoy this day that we've been given... Enjoy this day that we've been given..."

    Alone with Ini, I looked to perceive Qi over her casket; connecting with her energy, it directed me outwards, slowly spinning me around to enjoy the beautiful yellow leaves on the mulberry tree and the ripe orange fruit of the mandarin tree, so to suggest a message, "It's OK to turn away from death and enjoy the things of life."

    The energy grew stronger, beaming outwards with the same message in my head, "It's OK to turn away from death and go towards the things of life."

    Even when my most beautiful, wonderful daughter was in the casket, with whom I have so many memories... for whom I treated essentially every moment with love, and, for sure, she treated me every day with love... It seemed OK to enjoy and appreciate the beautiful things of life in this world.

    It's OK for me to move on and move forward.

    And take those beautiful. wonderful memories of her with me...

CHAPTER EIGHTY-EIGHT

That which brings life...

Returning to the casket, I attempted to perceive Ini's energy again... Same result – Gently pushed outwards into the natural world: This great tree with its beautiful yellow leaves that I love. Our mandarin tree. It is time for me to go out into the world and embrace life.

That is what Ini's spirit wants me to do, I thought. And that I will honor. Take her with me everywhere. Because love is Ini. Because love is that which brings life...

CHAPTER EIGHTY-NINE

Voice in my head…

Following the Qi emitted from Ini's casket yet another time, the energy again moved outwards, and appreciating the leaves on the trees and the fruit on the branches, I also felt directed towards our cars.

I wondered why this would be? Was it to appreciate all the drives we had made together with Ini?

Then, I noticed that, as compared to the Acura, the registration for the Subaru was expired.

Checking the Subaru's glove compartment, I found I did have the registration tag for the Subaru, but just hadn't put it on the license plate.

When I consider doing this, I felt conflicted, being that we had plans to return Ini to the morgue shortly, so that I might only have a few more minutes with her.

Then, a feminine voice spoke in my head.

"Take care of the things of the world, sweet boy," it said. "It's time."

I felt it was Ini's spirit… Just in her new form…

I questioned what I was hearing; though, later, I'd find I'd hear that voice again.

It was while I was trying to eat the chicken breast I'd made for Ini the night before (and had gone un-eaten), and I didn't want to let it go to waste, especially as I was hungry.

But I felt a terrible wave of nausea, given that the chicken had been meant for Ini, and she was no longer with us.

I tried to look on the bright side, thinking, "Perhaps the nausea will help me lose weight?"

Then, I heard that feminine voice again.

"Mike," it said, "maybe you give yourself a break and let go of your father's ways..."

CHAPTER NINETY

"Power animal..."

Standing at Ini's casket again between April and her mother, the movement of the energy that I perceived was slow; it started with a feeling of energy in my hands that directed my hands upwards till activating my crown chakra.

I thought the energy was only going to be directed my way; however, then the energy directed my hands outwards to both April and her mother, as they reported the activation of their crown chakra's.

Then, the energy directed my hands to my chest, and I felt my lungs expand, though not very much, so that I was afraid I was not going to share much healing to the others. However, after a couple of passes with me going from my chest to their chest areas, back and forth, it did seem that I became an effective channel for them, as April perceived a lot of warmth at her chest, and her mother also felt a sense of relief at her chest.

"Thank you, Ini," April said.

"Thank you, spirit of Ini," her mother added.

It struck me that for the rest of my life I was going to have to say...

"There's Ini energy," April's mother completed for me.

Yes, I had a spirit animal helper now. Like beyond Qi Gong, there was a native healing element to it.

Because I think that Ini was going to be sending healing energy through me to others for the rest of my life.

133

"Wonderful," April's mother said. "She's your power animal now..."

CHAPTER NINETY-ONE

Lamentation...

Rather than return Ini to the morgue, we decided to keep her with us overnight. Despite being in the casket, April insisted we put Ini in the garage, so to keep her safe from animals that might feed on her.

During the night, April lamented Ini's passing.

"Even with all of our resources and knowledge and education," she began, "in the past three or four weeks it was worthless to help our daughter. All we could do was try to get her yummy meat, which we knew wasn't the best thing for her. But it was the only thing in our power... It was all we could do.

"But it was also hopeless... We were helpless. All these resources, all the money that we had, all the medical knowledge that we had, our ability to go to people who could do something about it, and everybody just said, 'It can't be helped... There's no help.'

"So, all we could do was love her and hold her and comfort her. That was all we could do."

And she wanted to be there for us, I said, because she loved us so much, and she loved life so much, so to endure so much suffering.

And she taught me a lesson: That even with all of my knowledge and experience - medical, spiritual - I could still be brought to my knees and traumatized by the agony of feeling I'd failed a beloved being.

Who could imagine what it is for people who didn't have our resources? I asked. How they feel?

"I did fail when it came to her fatigue," April confided. "She was already doing some of that thing where she'd go into that deep, deep,

deep sleep. She was already starting to show some of that. Which meant she had been sick for a long time…

"And we were going to doctors… And they didn't see it."

Yes, we were all blindsided, I said. It just didn't make sense: How do you get a dog through one cancer concern to be followed by another? Nobody wanted to consider that - Not even her oncologist.

"Until we got her to the UC Davis emergency room," April concluded, "and finally somebody said, 'It sounds like cancer…'"

CHAPTER NINETY-TWO

Regrets...

"At least we had those three weeks to show her how much we loved her," April continued. "If only I could have done more with her the month earlier when she was functional. It was all, 'Facial scar! Facial scar! Blah blah blah."

This referring to the laceration to her forehead after tripping on Ini's dog ramp on Halloween.

"'Have to stay out of the sun,'" she continued. "So, I didn't spend my days in the park. I'm so sad about that."

She cried...

CHAPTER NINETY-THREE

"Blinded..."

"We were all blinded," April continued. "I was blinded. I thought that she got better: She was just a finicky eater - Weight loss was good for her – Good for her joints."

"But the fatigue and weight loss," she added. "I failed her..."

CHAPTER NINETY-FOUR

Potentially worse...

I listened to April – though, really, I thought having not found the cancer early was all a blessing: If we had caught it earlier, we might have put her through chemotherapy for the cancer, which I contend would have just made matters worse and would have tortured her.

April commented about how it was that a nephew was contending with a severe exacerbation of an autoimmune condition and how was currently felt that the diagnostic procedures run had made the condition worse.

In turn, my mind drifted to what neurology attendings had told me about procedures to evaluate neurologic conditions before there was MRI - How they would send contrast material into the cerebral spinal fluid, from the base of the spine all the way into the ventricles of the brain to look and see what was going on in the nervous system, which would often provoke a Chemical neuritis; that is, literally a chemical burn of the nerves from the spine to the brain, all the way through.

Listening to these old-time neurologists talk about this, I wondered how they could live with themselves after having seen reactions like that in response to their diagnostic endeavors? What they had caused in an attempt to figure out what their patients had and how it was worse than the disease. How did they live with themselves. They'd basically given someone the equivalent of what Ini suffered with the GME...

CHAPTER NINETY-FIVE

Soft look even after...

April recalled some of the ironies in Ini's lab results compared to what we'd been watching on the ground.

"The fact that she was so dehydrated," April said. "Even when she was drinking a river and then passing urine through that diseased organ of hers every hour. Just driven to using that organ. Just drink, drink, drink, drink and still be thirsty."

So, in the end we gave her some ease.

"And we lost a being who cared for us."

But even from the great beyond.

"She's still with us in her energy."

And giving to us perhaps because we cared for her.

"Yes, we cared. We loved her..."

And perhaps we helped showed her the way... To heaven?

Those last moments that she was looking into my eyes, my Crown chakra popped, so perhaps to help facilitate a direct connection with the universal Chi, the divine energy of the universe, that she now seemed to be sending back to us.

"How else did she have such a soft look in her eyes, so to make me able to pet her dead body for eight hours," April commented. "I mean, I gets so icked out by dead bodies. I get horrified. And I was petting and interacting with her, and it was because she just looked so peaceful and cute, with her doll and just that look of hers."

"And that was the look that she was giving you," she asserted. "It was such a comfort to have that look."

April kissed me.

"Thank you," she whispered. "Thank you..."

CHAPTER NINETY-SIX

"Too hard..."

I reflected on how hard this life could be on people and God's creatures.

"Yeah, that's my problem," April responded. "With Him. I've had that problem for a while now... The past five years.... Then I fell into Renewal, and I was chanting, and I really felt the energy, and it was really meaningful to me; but then we got the hit with Ini, and it was like, "God, you make things too hard."

"I mean, if there really is an intelligence that created all this... There's something sadistic..."

CHAPTER NINETY-SEVEN

"Just struggle..."

"From a very young age," April continued. "I had a problem with the whole 'eating' thing."

That is, most every living thing eats another living thing.

"And people tell me," she added, 'That's how the cycle of life works. Renewal of resources. Old things die and get consumed by young things. And that there's a beauty to that.... As a way to continue life.'

"But I still see all of that suffering and say, 'This is too much, God.' And I mean, if You're creating something, why not make it so at some point the creatures go, 'OK, that's my time and now I need to give my turn to someone else, and I'm really happy about doing that.' Why keep that fear of death? Why not give a, 'Wow! I had my turn. It was so great. Here, I want to have someone else have a turn.' Why couldn't He have created that and handed that to the cycle of life?

"This suffering is there, and I don't get why it has to be there? And why He didn't create us all with a different end stage that we move to, with less fear and suffering around it? By having us be born with a different attitude about it

"At some point our biological clock goes, 'Ding dong', time to move on to the next plane. And it's a wonderful thing. Or at least, it's not a terrible thing."

"It doesn't seem like He gave that to anybody or anything," she concluded. "Instead, it's just struggle..."

CHAPTER NINETY-EIGHT

God's shining example...

I nodded.

I was true: Ini was such a perfect specimen of love and God's creation. And yet, when it came to the idealistic ways that a perfect creation would respond to opening up space for another, even she didn't fall in line?

"I think it's a critical cruelness in the design of this world," April responded. "I've talked about this with a couple of rabbis and more enlightened people than me... About me feeling bad from the time that I was a kid about the world and why I have a hard time with being religious... And people have tried to get me to see that there's a beauty in the cycles and the renewability of life that one being uses their physical body for a time... And then some other organism uses the resources to have their own body and life, and that there's a beauty to that.

"But it's cruel that that process demands pain, suffering, loss and horror involves giving up the resources that life requires."

I asserted that it seemed to me that she was asking for a certain degree of rationality and logic from beings, and it might be that there's a reason for emotion? That love, in the case of Ini, wants to hold on. And love, in the case of me, wants to let go, so that she can go to God and not continue suffering.

And that emotion is what makes us spirit entities, and not simply machines.

We are more than machines... We love.

And there's a price to pay for having this gift of being able to love.

And pain is part of that price.

It's the price we pay for the gift of love.

It's just like the Lakota say, every gift comes with a sacrifice. It shouldn't just all be for free.

"So, my own personal sacrifice for the past five years involve my hair.... Well, it actually involved a lot more than that.... And I have to tell you it's so nice to have it shorter. It's light, fluffy and it doesn't get in the way. Even though my hair got a lot thinner over the years, it was so heavy to have that much hair. and it got tangled and knotted all the time.

"So, on some level, I've been ready to cut my hair for a while. It doesn't mean I wanted to. But it was a sacrifice on my part."

I consider the sacrifices that Ini made to be alive these past five years.: To fight through pain that I'm sure I would never be able to imagine with that GME.

"Yeah, and we kept wanting to have her more lucid, so we didn't give her as much gabapentin to reduce her pain," she responded. "But, also, she just hated to be pilled every day."

It seemed to me that Ini struggled because she loved us so much. If the purpose of life is to learn about love on the fiscal plane, it seemed that Ini's life certainly afforded an example of that.

And to the point of a willingness to give up your turn and go gracefully into the next life... Well, it seemed to me that that thing that mostly went you go 'Ding dong' was the pain of life... That's what seemed to leave a lot of my patients feeling like, 'OK, it's time for me to check out. It's time for me to let somebody else have their turn.' Because when the pain of life becomes too much, then it's time.

But, in the words of Albert Ellis, we 'f'd up, fallible human beings' aren't totally sure what there is after this life. So, we hold on to this one... Because we're scared.

Even I'm scared... And I know better than most what it feels like to nearly die... And what there is during this life:

When I was a boy of about ten, I was playing in the ocean when I was pulled under by a wave and caught in an undertow. Tossed and unable to reach the surface, I surrendered: To this day I can still recall taking in the water; however, also in that moment, I experienced a feeling of serenity like none I'd ever known before or since – and I think that was my endorphin system kicking in, to help me conserve what was left of my oxygen resources before a lifeguard pulled me out...

In the end, it seems to me that whatever God or this divine energy is... Well, even if Its intention was as perfect as April wanted... Well, as someone who helped develop a cancer vaccine, it's my experience that, between the intention and the developing of something, there's a lot of trial and error; and it could be that we're still in that development phase, and God and the divine energy are still working to figure it out (You know... Evolution).

Hence, maybe He/She isn't doing the worst job. Because even though all of us organisms have these anatomical and physiological processes that go wrong, we're still all built with self-destruct mechanisms, as well as an overwhelming stress responses, whereby when we're stressed beyond the limit of our endurance, essentially every organism on the planet is able to enter a suspended state of animation called the freeze response - Which I experienced firsthand when I nearly drowned, and it produced the best feeling of my life.

But when I came back to "land of the living", I think I got so invested in wanting to live so badly that I got terrified about being put in a compromising situation again... Perhaps because then the cerebral cortex kicks in, and there's doubt, and the question, "What if there isn't something else out there?", etc., and you wind up hanging on to life, and in my case, developing a fear of air hunger, so you have difficulty putting yourself into even a sauna or a sweat lodge.

"My feeling was similar," April responded. "And while you were performing Qi Gong, I had my eyes closed, And it was allowing me to open up and talk about everything, all my fears, and where talking with Anna and Dan [friends] was so healing to me and pumped up my endorphins, so that I was feeling good; but then I walked to the back and I was confronted with Ini's coffin, And I started thinking about things, and my mind went to horror. So that it was like, 'Oh, I could take a moment to really enjoy myself, but then my mind went to what we had experienced on Thursday and Friday, and the total loss; so that I was feeling like, 'How can it be?'"

She broke down and cried.

"It's such a substantial loss. All the little things. All the little joys. The little knock on the door when we're talking with each other, and you look out and it's Ini wanting to join us; And it's like, 'Oh, this being wants to be a part of us, interacting with each other'; or checking up on me while I'm in the bathroom; or just walking around the house, I can hear her paws and I'm like, 'Oh, I think I know where Ini is... That's Ini... Ini walking around the house'; Or when she decides to join us in bed, and comes and jumps in here... She just wanted to be with us... She wanted us to be happy."

Yes, a being who loved us unconditionally, who just offered us all of the healthy, functional pleasures in life... A walk out into nature, experiencing all the beauty in life.

"Or bring you a toy and be like, 'Time to play... Time to get out of the house... What are you doing in the house all this time? There's beautiful stuff outside.'"

Just all of that simple goodness in a life that could seem so complicated.

"Yeah, you see a problem and you try to come up with some solution; and that ends up causing this problem... And you try to address that problem, and something else happens."

I think we are still evolving; and we get really good at some things, but other things we're not so good at yet (like Ini's aggressive cancer). So, we're brought down to our knees...

In any event, it seemed to me that perhaps God wasn't Almighty in effecting the perfect design from the start. Nevertheless, I'd like to think the intention of the universe is good and driven by love.

And to build something that's just love... Well, it seemed to me that that was no easy task. It takes time and work and trial and error. As they say, invention was one percent inspiration and 99% perspiration.

And perhaps we spirits are sent into the physical plane to become a part of that developmental process, and we do as well as we can with our physical bodies, but they are not perfect.

And if you ask me, Ini was as close a shining example of the kind of being that April was talking about as could have been created; because through all of those physical problems, she essentially maintained most of those precepts that April was looking for – except maybe the one about conceding it was her time to go

But, even there (and I rather hate to admit this), I'm not all that sorry she wasn't so inclined to give up her space to another when it was her time; I rather like and appreciate the fact that she wanted to be with us in spite of all her suffering. In retrospect, it leaves me feeling really loved.'..."

CHAPTER NINETY-NINE

"Channeling Ini..."

During the night, I had a vision of the silhouette of a physically attractive woman dressed in black and moving cat-like in the garage.

We had placed Ini in the garage during the night to protect her from any scavengers that might go after her physical remains.

So, I wasn't scared; and had the feeling that this was a spirit related to Ini.

In the morning, though, when I opened the door adjoining the house and the garage, Cat Chow came running in.

She had been with Ini all night; and, more than that, I had the feeling that the spirits of these two animals were communing with each other.

April had been very impressed with Cat Chow, who, just now, jumped into bed, as though "channeling Ini", by wanting to lay down with us.

"She cared about Ini, and Ini cared about us," April said. "And now she's like, 'Mom and dad are talking to each other. I better come in and be a part of it.'"

Yes, just like Ini would, I thought...

But I don't trust Cat Chow, I countered. I don't think she can be as selfless as Ini.

And whereas Ini never got angry at me, I think Cat Chow can.

And whereas Ini would rather die than disappoint me, Cat Chow can act out.

And, hence, here I am, spoiling this wonderful moment with Cat Chow because she isn't Ini.

But such is grief and mourning, I thought. And God help me that I may one day come to a place that I'll accept a being that's less than perfect (like Cat Chow) and appreciate and embrace her – like Ini accepted me...

CHAPTER ONE HUNDRED

Enduring energy...

We went looking to test if items associated with Ini (like her paw prints and previously shed hair) might elicit the effect of promoting a healing experience by starting with perceiving energy from these objects.

And it was very interesting that the moment I perceived energy over the hair and paw prints, the energy went into my other hand and then seemed to be sending energy over to April at her midline chakras, before going down her body and into the ground, and then up to the top of my head, to create a strong feeling at my crown chakra, until I felt this strong, tight beam between my crown chakra and the universal Chi; and then it went back to April and did the same thing, such that this object created this amazing circuit between April and myself and mother earth and the universal Chi!

So, I'd say these objects are eliciting the same kind of a fact that starting with Ini's remains did.

"My headache is very reduced," April added. "It felt different than your usual bioenergy. Like it wasn't exactly from the body itself."

No, it was coming from an enduring energy that was initiated from Ini...

CHAPTER ONE HUNDRED AND ONE

Last session...
Sunday, December 24, 2023

We took a walk to the park, traveling the way we usually would with Ini. Within the park, April encountered some of our 'dog friends' and spent some time chatting with them. I, on the other hand, just wanted to be alone with my thoughts and stood in the center of the tennis court surveying the land (like looking out at the Plains) and dictating the past days events into my voice recorder, and feeling so uncomfortable in my body, my back and shoulders aching everywhere.

Returning to the house, we entered the backyard, where Ini was, and in the presence of April and her mother (Ima), I looked to perceive energy from over Ini's casket.

Unlike the other times, it took a long time before I perceived a directionality to it and it would initiate movement. Before that, it was holding me, but in a very subtle form.

Finally, it generated some movement, bending me low towards the ground, before finally sending my arms in the direction of April (across from me) and Ima to my left.

And then I felt energy being sent from my hands, but in a very different way than Chi has ever been sent from my hands before: Instead of feeling the energy move outwards from my palms (hands perpendicular to my arms), it was being sent through my outstretched fingers (which were parallel with my arms).

And they were strong beams of energy that were being sent out from me.

Then, the energy bent me low again and directed my arms outwards – though this time only towards April (again, across from me) with energy beaming out the same way as before; that is, not from my palms, but like beams coming out from my outstretched fingers that were parallel with the rest of my arms.

Then, the energy directed me to stand up straight, and it was 'over.' There was a feeling like my sweet doggie was saying, "You don't need my body. You have all the tools and objects and momentos you need. Lay me to rest in any way you want, and you go on with what you have, without carrying me or exhuming me.

And the lingering impression I got from this 'ceremony' was it felt 'holy.' Like it was more than Qi I was dealing with. That this was pertaining to the spirit. Like performing someone's last rites.

It was a very deep experience - different from anything I had ever experienced before. It was slow and deliberate and took a long time. The energy was very subtle while I was following it, and then very strong when it finally beamed out from me...

CHAPTER ONE HUNDRED AND TWO

Parting gift...

Stepping back from Ini's casket, I shared with the others what I'd experienced and that there was no working with Ini this way again.

April became animated, imploring me to please attempt it another time, saying that in spite of the deep and intense experience I had, she hadn't been imparted with the feeling she was anticipating.

But I had to tell her that I couldn't – There was something I couldn't disavow – That I'd experienced a deeper, more solemn, serious feeling of awe and reverence than I'd ever felt before while connecting energetically, and I had to honor that feeling by respecting that this was the last time.

And as I was imparting this to her, my body was literally transforming right there were I stood – Going from a state in which I was uncomfortable in it, to a state in which I felt incredibly grounded - And this essentially right after we had been in the park, and I had been dictating in the tennis courts, and I was feeling so uncomfortable in my body – Probably less than an hour ago! Now, here I was so comfortable in my body and feeling like I was standing strong! I literally felt powerful.

I took a step and felt grounded and balanced, so to contribute to the feeling of strength.

Looking at April quizzically, she acknowledged that she could see it, too.

"You're standing straighter," she commented...

Feeling like I wanted to be in nature, I walked towards the river.

Then, as I entered the fields, my friend, Sam, called, and I told him about the last energy experience with Ini's body in the casket, and especially this amazing feeling of strength and being grounded; and unlike all the other times I'd ever spoken with him about matters that might touch on something spiritual, this time he was willing to comment.

"We haven't figured out what work Ini has to do in that other life," he began. "But she has to move on. She has other things and other places that she has to take care of that we can't even imagine.

"And so, my feeling is, that's it - Ini is now gone.

"But the last thing she wanted to do was to give you this before she left - That is, totally left.

"So, I think you have to honor that, like you're saying. I think you figured it out - That you're honoring it, because you're not going to get anything else out of it – Except memories of good times - And that's all that's going to sustain you.

"It's like I can't keep demanding things from my dad who has passed away… Or my grandfather, or my grandmother, or my aunts, or my uncles. Unless, somehow, they reach over and touch you. Then, you have to be receptive to that, I guess. I don't know, I've never felt that.

"But it's like the saying, 'God helps those who help themselves' - You have to really put in effort. It's up to you. She's given you some tools to give you a little bit of an advantage, as a last resort - Now it's up to you to take it on.

"Because you're just going to get older and more damaged; but for now, she saying, 'Hey, enjoy your life a little bit more right now.'

"So, I think that you should accept it and make the best out of it.

"And she's probably also saying, 'There may be another dog in your life? You might meet another creature that's alive and give you great aid and comfort.' But she's done everything she can while she was alive, and now she's got to move on."

My thoughts drifted to April, who said that in all of the other sessions, she had felt the energy coming from my work at Ini's casket, but at this time she did not, and this despite the strong energy that seem to be coming from my hands towards her in this different way that Energy had ever been sent from me before?

"I don't understand that, either," Sam said. "I can only say to take what you have, and that's been given to you, and move on. Because I think Ini probably knows that there's another dog or animal or creature that needs you (just like she needed you), so that now you have to move on, and Ini has moved on, as well - And I don't think you're going to feel much more from it.

I confided that the scientist in me wanted to go back and test this again; but the inner core of me said, No - This with everything that this being had. And you have to honor that.

"Yeah, because you're dealing with a live being," he responded, "and it's not something that you can experiment with."

"Like anything," he added, "you can only dissect something so many times - and that's it. it's not the same.

"So, I don't think you want to go there. Because what you'll find is things that won't deliver any usefulness.... It's just now become just like anything else. It's an element. It's gone down to the elemental level. I'm sure you can keep going and take it down to an electron. But it's the same darn electron found in everything. So that all you've done is dissect it down and down and down till you've lost Ini - and it's just organic matter that everything contains.

"And that's not what you're after: you were after Ini.

"But Ini has left. She is gone.

"So now, I think you have to accept Ini's parting gift, but she's also taught you that there's something even until the very end - So when you do Qi Gong to a person as they're closing in on their final moments of existence, you're going to be able to feel it more - Because you felt it with Ini - before and after."

I confided to Sam about how I'd been dictating in the tennis court just an hour ago, feeling so uncomfortable in my body and thinking, "I have to get back to acupuncture. I have to get back to working on my body. I'm so uncomfortable in my body." This was literally just an hour ago when April and I were taking a walk in the park before we did this last Qi Gong over Ini's casket, and, after doing that, and talking with April and telling her I didn't think that I could do this again, this transformation happened... Which was a long way of saying that it strikes me that I don't need acupuncture, or trigger point therapy or electrostimulation... Everything is simply already there.

"Right," he responded. "But don't think it's permanent. No gift lasts forever.

"So, you just need to enjoy it - Ini wants you to be happy right now. She wants you to feel good about her, about you, about the world around you, your environment, and so she's giving you that. Can you ask for a better gift than that? No, you can't. You can't. You can't.

"So, just accept it, and use it while you can, until it disappears."

Nevertheless, it seems to be telling me, "Mike, you are OK in your body. Your problem is energy disturbances, and you can get better."

"Right, but let's talk about this in a week or a month and see where you're at?" Sam responded.

"I guess what I'm saying is," he added, "Don't blame Ini if things start to fade. Because even Ini doesn't have that capability - But she gave everything she could to you from what she could.

"And you can only give what you can. So, like I say, enjoy it, because it's a gift that you'll probably never get again - You'll probably never get this strength or this type of quality of a gift ever again."

"You're discovering more about the mysteries of the universe," he asserted. "Kind of neat. You're in a special place. Not very many other people will have experience this.

"Some people have - People who have had a loved one pass away and all of the sudden made them realize that they made them a better person - For all those people, they perceive a very special gift.

"So, you're not the only one - But not everyone gets it, either.

"So, you just have to be very thankful. Thankful that Ini came into your life. And she left with such a very remarkable gift to you on her passing."

I confided that I was experiencing a sense of awe and reverence like I didn't think I ever had in my life.

"Well, I think you'll experience similar things more and more as you do your practice," he responded. "Because now you're more receptive to it, and you're more open to people and their generous capabilities and goodness."

He wished me a good time over Christmas and thanked me for all I had done over the past year.

"I'm sure I'll talk to you before New Year's," he concluded, "and we'll see what the New Year brings..."

Postscript

April would later comment that it wasn't just me who'd received a bodily parting gift from Ini.

"There was some kind of beginning of a process that happened that I noticed immediately," she said. "I don't think I had words for it on that day, but I understood it later. That it was probably a fascia thing. And I was suddenly more flexible. And that allowed me to do stuff that is continuing to make me more flexible! So, it's like it's continuing."

An enduring gift, I thought.

"I was very bound up before that," she continued. "It was almost like I was in bondage. And then it released. And it was some kind of release that allowed things to progress.

"And it was just like that. From one day to the next – Click! – And I didn't do anything.

"And I wasn't aware of it like you were. Like it happened to me, but I wasn't so quick to recognize it. I acknowledged it, but I didn't understand it. I didn't have words for it then.

"And maybe it was because I wasn't looking for something like that. I wasn't expecting anything like that. I was in so much grief. But then I suddenly felt free – in my body.

"So, I think it was different for me than it was for you. You were going after her energy and interacting with it, and I was along with you, and I was there with you, but I was more seeking..."

She broke off and her eyes welled up.

"I was more seeking more time with her," she add through her tears. "I wanted some kind of message. I wasn't looking for bodily healing or anything like that. I just wanted time that she still existed and could see me. And that she was OK. I just wanted to be with her a little bit longer..."

CHAPTER ONE HUNDRED AND THREE

Fatherly advice...

To my intense surprise, out of nowhere, my father called to say that he was concerned about what he been hearing about Ini.

I told him that I found that incredibly kind.

"Well, you'd do the same thing for me!" he responded.

I told him about the events on Thursday night: That at one in the morning, April observed labored breathing, by two in the morning we had her at the veterinarians, by three they had performed some tests, in particular, an arterial blood gas, and by four, we made the decision to euthanize her.

"Oh, that's really tough," he responded.

Yes, and it had shaken my spiritual beliefs, because instead of just slipping into the next life in a contented way, Ini was looking right into my eyes and indicating to me that she was OK with suffering, so that she could continue to be with me.

So, it really hurt to feel like I let my dog down by not honoring her request in those last moments.

"Well, I think that would be the same way any dog owner would react, Michael," he began. "And what you're experiencing is the most difficult part of having a pet... Because we know we're going to outlive them. And that day will come, and we have to make that very difficult decision as to how to prepare them for what we have to do to make the pain go away.

"And there is no easy choice... We have no choice.

"But we have to think of them, and not of us wanting to keep them alive for a little bit longer, another day, another week, another month. Because we don't know the pain that they're experiencing while we keep them alive.

"We've been through that with a number dogs that we've had and it's never, ever an easy decision to make when you know that the injection you're going to give them is going to put them out of any pain that they're ever going to feel.

"And we know that that's the right thing to do. We don't want them to die with a lot of pain and suffering that we can alleviate for them.

"And it's so difficult on everybody. But we want to do the right thing and we're not sure what is the real right thing to do. Can we keep them alive another week? Month? Year? But what happens during that week? Month? Year? Are they really enjoying life? Or are they having pain every time they get up to walk to come see you? It's the toughest thing an animal owner is facing when that time comes. But they have to get past that to realize they don't want to see their dog in pain.

"It's that dichotomy where they don't want to see their dog in pain and they don't want to see their dog put down.

"But they don't give us any choice. We have to do what's the most comfortable for our pet, and it's the hardest thing I think an owner has to take responsibility for with their pet.

"And we'll try every medication, every procedure that's available in order to try to keep them with us. But it may be to no avail and it's just a matter of wrenching it out a little longer. And when that happens, you have to ask, 'Are we being stingy?'

"We've had a number of dogs, and over the years, we've had to deal with this question. And it's never an easy answer.

"The right thing to do is to relieve them of the pain. But it's so hard to carry through.

"I mean, it's the hardest thing in the world for a pet owner to do. But we've got to think of them and not us - How do we make their last time with us somewhat pleasurable?

"I mean, Ini's been through a lot of different things that you've done to prolong and make her life comfortable. But there comes a point where you realize you're fighting a losing battle and it's only a matter of time.

"And that's OK - Because those last hours, days, whatever they have left are going to be important. To you and to your pet.

"So, you got to do the tough thing. And I know how hard it's going to be to do that. And haven't gone through it with a number of pets that we've had, it's never easy.

"It kills you to do that and tell the vet, 'Go ahead, put that needle in them and put them to sleep.'

"Believe me, I know exactly – exactly - everything that's going through your mind: 'Is there one thing I can do? Maybe I can try a new this or a new that?'

"But, inevitably , we run out of things we can do for them. And in a way, ridding them of the pain that they are experiencing is probably the most humane thing we really can do."

I told him that I felt it was amazing that a being could love you so much that they could want to stay with you in spite of intense suffering.

"Of course," he responded. "I understand completely. We've been through this ourselves a number of times and it is never, never, ever easy making that decision.

"But there comes a point where you don't want the dog to suffer.

"Are there miracle cures? Are there things tomorrow morning? Something you can do and she'll be perky and jumping all around another day? Well, believe me, I could never find one pill or the one Veterinarian who could give me more time. Instead, the time they do give you is no pleasure to your pet.

"It's hard, Mike. I sat there crying when the doctor brought out the needle that I knew was going to end their life.

"But I knew, rather than expose them to nothing more than pain and discomfort, it was time. It was the right thing to do.

"And I don't regret myself for ever doing it, Mike. Because I know how much pain they were going through, how much discomfort, how much they were trying to stay with us, but it was being selfish to keep them in that way.

"So, I'm not trying to make up your mind for you. You'll know, because she's been your lifelong friend, and you'll know what has to be done, and that time will come.

"But it doesn't make it any easier. Trust me, Mike. I know exactly what's going through your mind and the pain it's causing. And there's not much you or I can do to relieve that pain."

I expressed my gratitude for his call.

"Well, it's the least…"

He became overwhelmed.

"I'm sitting here crying," he managed. "It's the least I can do to tell you, having been through it a good number of times, it's never, ever easy to put down a pet. Never."

Just then, April indicated that there was something she wanted me to see.

"That's OK," my father said. "We'll catch up. We've got plenty to talk. We'll catch up. Honestly..."

What strikes me now is how obviously depressed my father must be. I have never heard him cry before. And this time he broke down.

And my father sounded like I never thought he would sound like again.

"Maybe the Ini energy went into him and gave you that gift of the father you never thought you were going to hear again," April said...

CHAPTER ONE HUNDRED AND FOUR

Last pawprint...

Leading me into the yard, April said she'd located a pawprint of Ini's.

There, by a tree where Ini used to lay, was an impression of Ini's paw that matched exactly a pawprint that April had made from clay!

Amazed at the discovery, I asked how she found it?

She responded that it had literally reached out to her and shone with golden light...

CHAPTER ONE HUNDRED AND FIVE

Without...

As April had not felt what she'd anticipated in that last Qi Gong experience over Ini's casket, I offered to perform Qi Gong with April and her mother in the usual way.

Doing this, I perceived Qi from April; she, in turn, reported she felt it in her heart, and then that energy extend it to her mother, so that both of them had an experience in which they felt "elevated."

And it just felt like it was time to do this without calling on Ini...

CHAPTER ONE HUNDRED AND SIX

Letting her rest...

Taking a walk with April to the river's edge (where I had taken one of April's favorite photos of she and Ini), April and I talked about letting Ini go after that Qi Gong session between she, her mother and me.

"Because as you can see with my room, I have a really hard time letting go," she said. "Even for stuff that has stopped being useful, I have a hard time letting go.

"So, when it came to Ini's remains... Well, that was an impossible mental state for me to get into."

I talked about my own difficulty, especially with that last Qi Gong experience over Ini's body and how it felt like it spoke to my ancestral roots as a Kohen, and the prohibition not to interact with the deceased.

"They have their own journey," April responded.

I continued that it felt like I could now understand the origins of the Jewish tradition to quickly bury these hosts of spiritual beings within a limited period of time. That there was a reason for it.

"Why?" she asked.

It just felt like I had this humbling experience involving the awesome nature of God, I said. And it called for a really deep and real respect. Like it was saying to me, "You don't call on this form...the deceased ...to continually work with you. It's time to let these mortal remains rest."

"That's why I had this intimate feeling that I should only take a tiny little bit of hair from Ini," she responded. "And when it was done, I couldn't take anymore. Or paw prints. I just had this respect and the idea that somehow interacting with her body or walking around with one of her bones… That felt so wrong.

"I know that the cremation people are going to say if we pay them, they can take more paw prints, and there are also digital paw prints. But I'm thinking that I want them to interact with her as little as possible. And I want them to manipulate her as little as possible.

"I mean, I was kind of intrigued with their digital paw prints… I was intrigued by having that. But at the same time, I felt I want to honor her and let her rest..."

CHAPTER ONE HUNDRED AND SEVEN

Another time...

"Do you think we'll meet her when we die?" April asked.

Yes, I had no doubt.

Indeed, I wondered what it might be like to meet her in her spirit form, in which she'd be our equal and not of a different species?

Indeed, I thought that would be a humbling day.

"Ini, keep your ears and eyes open for us," April said. "For when I come."

I thought Ini would be looking out for her for the rest of her life.

I told her if she wanted, we could do Qi Gong every day, applying Ini's paw prints and other items if she wanted.

"Oh, I'd love that," she responded.

"I think it's time," she said, indicating it was getting dark. "I think the wild is beginning to look at us."

We sang the Lakota prayer song and other songs as we made our way home...

CHAPTER ONE HUNDRED AND EIGHT

Conclusion – "…good and powerful…"

Arriving back at the house, we sang more prayer songs as we prepared to bring Ini back to the morgue.

I shared what Dan Foster had told me about Lakota culture; that was, for those born with disabilities, these were individuals who were honored by the members of the tribe, because they were regarded as embodied by spirits that were willing to come into this world in a really challenge state so to live this lifetime; and for that, they honor that person.

And considering how much Ini has suffered through her life, with a leg fracture and GME and now this very aggressive form of cancer, I think she had earned her place in really being honored…

In the backyard April pointed out a 6-inch plank some 3 feet above the ground against the fence.

"Do you remember when Ini would jump up here and then chase squirrels back-and-forth?" she asked. "We used to use this backyard a lot more before that knee surgery."

Yes, the surgery before Ini acquired GME.

"Ini, I don't believe you need this body anymore," she said over the casket. "Or, at least, I hope you don't need this body anymore."

"It gave you a lot of pleasure," she added.

Yes, and it gave me pleasure – To watch her with all that agility, dexterity and grace. She could turn on a dime and out race me anytime!

"But it also gave you a lot of pain," April declared. "And I, for one, hope you have a situation without being painful, and you can do everything you want to do."

167

"And your dad thinks that you're good and powerful now," she concluded. "And I want that for you, too..."

EPILOGUE

Within a few months of Ini's passing, our dear friend and neighbor, Beth, passed away suddenly and unexpectedly.

April revisited the events of Beth's syncopal episode when she shared her passing with our 'spirit buddy', Steve.

"When Mike finally got Beth out of the car, she was very disoriented, so that we called for the ambulance and Mike ultimately took her to the hospital. Then, she went through a lot of different tests... From what I understand, they didn't know quite what was going on with her... They were looking at her heart and they were looking at her brain... And because of everything that was going on with us, I wasn't having close contact with her, but our neighbors were following up with her...

"And me and my mom credited how much Ini cared about Beth for the fact that she kind of 'woke up.'

"Because Ini was fading... And then she woke up - and she ran. She was all puffed up, and then she had Monday and Tuesday, where she was like her old self. We walked to the park. She was interested in squirrels.

"Then, on Wednesday, we didn't make it all the way to the park. And then on Thursday, she could hardly walk. And then on Friday morning, we did the euthanasia.

"But, still, I'm convinced that the reason we even had that Monday and Tuesday was because somehow Ini cared about what happened to Beth so much that she somehow came back from the death process..."

April and I talked about that warm summer day when I met Beth: There I was walking with Ini by this house where behind the fence was the biggest German shepherd I had ever seen. This was the shark of dogs.

And I didn't have Ini on a leash because that was our way; that is, she came to me from the wild and I tried to respect that; on the Indian lands of the Northern Plains where fate brought us together and where we would walk together, she never required a leash and would simply come back to me when called, no matter how far away; and then, when she developed the chronic, persistent autoimmune meningitis, she always had lingering pain in her neck and spine, so that a leash or harness was painful for her.

So, there we were walking past the house that belonged to this really big German Shepherd. And I'm just feeling like I want to get past this house/dog and expecting my little dog to feel the same way (After all, Ine was all of 40 or 50 pounds).

Then, to my complete and utter surprise, I hear this shrill voice calling out to me, "Hey, your dog just shat on my yard."

I went running back, apologizing profusely, declaring that I couldn't imagine in my life that my dog would go pooping in the yard with such a big strong dog there...

"Afterwards," April commented, "Beth shared that Liam never let any other dog poop or pee on his lawn. Ini was the only dog that he let do that.

"Then, he would go and sniff it afterwards, and they would like exchange 'letters' that way. I would call them boyfriend and girlfriend.

"And then after Liam passed away, Beth told me, 'Well, I know that Liam liked Ini to go on my lawn, but now that he's gone, I don't want her to go on my lawn.'

"And I had a really hard time keeping Ini from doing that, because it was her habit. So, I actually started going on the other side of the street or doing all sorts of things. And Beth noticed that and said, 'You know what?... She could be the only dog to go on my lawn. Liam gave her permission and now I give her permission.'"

Liam was euthanized sometime after he developed a paralytic illness affecting his lower limbs (degenerative myelopathy). Before that, Beth had to put him in a harness in order to walk him.

My enduring memory of Liam was with Ini walking beside him and turning my head back in time to see the two of them sharing a kiss as they walked side-by-side.

"And shortly thereafter, he went..." April said...

April went to Beth's house to talk with Beth's sister (who inherited the house) to let her know about Liam's remains.

"I showed her a picture of Ini's urn, because it was just like Liam's," April said, "and let her know that it was Beth's wish that Liam's remains be spread over the island by the river, just like their father was."

April even went into the house and looked for the urn, but didn't find it, and wasn't willing to go through Beth's belongings to locate it.

"I tried to find it, she said. "But they didn't know me, and I was in the house, and it was all kind of awkward.

"Still, I tried really hard to see if I could see it. They actually let me walk into two different rooms. But I drew the line at opening any drawers.

"The reason I showed them the picture of Ini's urn was because we chose the same urn for any that Liam had."

April continue that although Liam was a 'boyfriend', Ini actually had a 'harem.'

"She had another dog for whom they were boyfriend and girlfriend, at the same time as Liam," April said. "I mean, Liam was a really big German shepherd. And the other one was a really big, heavy pitbull."

"So, she had a type," she asserted. "She liked the bad boys. If Ini was a human daughter, she would have brought home a lot of burly biker types..."

Upon my mother's passing, April commented that if we were to name the year like native peoples did in their "winter counts", she'd called it, "The winter of many goodbyes."

"But then, I don't know if I want to call it 'good-byes'," she inserted, "because they weren't 'good'-byes... They were bye's. They weren't good."

"I think in Hebrew," she added, "I would more call it, 'The winter of 'gardot'... The approximate translation is 'separations.' If I were to be poetic, then it would be, 'The winter of many tears' or 'The time of many rips - Ripping.'"

"What would be the word that you would use?" she asked.

The winter of many partings, I responded.

"Ini," she began. "Rose [my mother], Robert [April's best friend], House [our landlord asked us to leave, so that he could have his daughter live there], Yale [at the last minute, they indicated they weren't going to let me teach BioEnerQi, so I declined their position]."

I added Marty Fulbright to the list of names, who was my best friend in Tennessee and had essentially saved my medical career twenty years ago.

"I forgot about Marty," April said. "He was the first."

"And now Cat Chow is winking," she added.

Cat Chow had been diagnosed with a recurrence of her lung cancer and been given a few months to live.

But, alas, in spite of all this, I contended that this had been a winter of many gifts.

The parting gift had been bestowed upon me energetically by Ini. The parting gift my mother bestowed was also energetic.

"Yeah, your mom certainly gave us a lot of gifts," April exclaimed. "Oh my God..."

Arriving home, Cat Chow was waiting on the chair in the front of the house.

"I wonder how she is going to take to all of the changes coming up?" April asked.

I thought of what my friend, Ben, would say – "The only thing you can count on is change..."

At the half-year mark following Ini's passing, April asked if I still see Ini the same way that haunted me the night that she died, looking to God, as though pleading to stay with us?

I said yes, but that I felt more reconciled that it had to be that way; that is, it had to be hard for Ini. Because it's supposedly said that all of those who truly are put on this earth to attain the highest level of enlightenment have to suffer a hard death. It's one of the trials and travails that they have to go through, so to take that next step in whatever soul journey they're on. Like Pinocchio becoming a 'real boy', it seems that to reach nirvana, you have to be willing to show total and unconditional love in the face of suffering.

So, it was just Ini's fate from the beginning that this is what awaited her. It was a part of her destiny – To show total and unconditional love in the face of agony.

It was the same way with my beloved friend, Ethel: She had pancreatic cancer (known to be associated with the worst pain known to Medicine) an she would have fought through anything... Any pain, any suffering... to have stayed there with her grandchildren and with us. She never wanted to leave us.

And when I shared that with someone, they told me, "Yes, that's the path of the enlightened ones. They have to go through that travail and trial."

So, it gives me some comfort to feel like it was just a part of Ini's destiny.

April indicated that she was doing better with the issue of grief and Ini.

"We were so blessed," she said.

That we were.

And I contend that we still are, I asserted, as I looked over at Cat Chow, who was sitting there next to Ini's urn.

"Yes, she loves us," April agreed. "In a cat way..."

April commented that she had been gifted with a couple of things by Ini.

"Like when you had your strengthening thing," she said, "I had a loosening of my stiffness. And it continues. I'm continuing to loosen up and become more flexible.

"And my hair got body and curls now. I'm so happy. I mean, I liked it straight how it was, but I'm finding I'm really loving all of this body. I never had that before..."

As I'd alluded to, April had purchased all kinds of DNA evaluation kits to determine Ini's lineage, but never wound up using any of them.

When I asked why she hadn't, she said it was because the incentive and motivation for those kits was so she could identify a dog to get like Ini in the future; however, then she decided against that when she learned something like that was much less than full proof.

"This one couple with a lot of money love their dog," April said. "So, after the dog died, they cloned it, and ended up with two puppies. And neither one of those puppies had the same personality as the original.

"Also, both the clones were different. So even though all three dogs were genetically identical, they all had different personalities.

"So, isn't that incredible that three different dogs with the same DNA all had different personalities? And two of them had gone through everything together - The same birthmother, the same pregnancy, the same puppyhood?"

It depends on the spirit, I asserted...

My mother-in-law related that she was following the Facebook page of a group that rescued dogs on the Indian Reservation where we'd acquired Ini.

"And every so often, there's a dog that sort of looks like and reminds me of Ini," she said.

"You and April had said that there were a number of strays on the Reservation," she continued. "And because you saved Ini when you did, she had a good life. So, I was very impressed that there was this rescue group that actually drives around and looks for strays."

And I was very impressed that she'd made the effort to search out and find such a group.

"And what they do that I love," she added, spiritedly, "is they show before and after pictures…. What they look like before they rescue the dog, and what they look like a week or so later."

She read me a blogpost about a recent rescue, and, listening, I was filled with thoughts of longing for the life we knew there…

The week marking a year since Ini's passing, April had gone back to the house and collected yellow leaves from the big Mulberry tree that Ini had been so intent on being outside with during her last days.

"I thought I'd get some and preserve them," she said. "There weren't that many leaves left and they were all wet because of the rain. So, I put them out to dry on the floor under the table, and they became all dry and crinkly. And then, when I was in the bathroom, I heard this rustling in them. So that when I opened the door, Cat Chow was there, lying on top of them! It was like she was saying, 'Oh, Ini's leaves! I know what to do with them. They are to play with.'

"She was totally jumping into them and making lots of noise. It was fun to watch. Just loving this pile of leaves."

"The leaves that are in good shape, I'm putting in a bowl around Ini's urn," she concluded. "But I kind of like it that Cat Chow plays in them first…"

At the time, I was struggling with an acute COVID infection, and Cat Chow had been a constant companion, insisting on being in bed with me throughout my illness (This to April's chagrin and consternation, being that cats can acquiree COVID).

Ini was the one who would usually insist on being with me when I was ill. But Cat Chow had more than risen to the occasion.

Indeed, April reminded me that Cat Chow has proved quite empathic and recounted the story about how it was that just before Ini passed, Cat Chow went into some crazed state, leaping up the apple tree in front of our house and then getting stuck there.

"She was having a hard time climbing down," April recalled, "so you went and helped her down the tree."

"She obviously knew," April continued, weeping. "She could sense Ini slipping away.

"And then she wouldn't go outside for two months. She just wouldn't go outside..."

As I've shared, Cat Chow has cancer, and we don't know how long she has.

But that certainly doesn't seem to bother her, as she appears a lot more focused on living.

Of note, just as I was feeling like I was coming out of COVID (before I got hit with COVID rebound), I was enjoying some live music being played at the end of an Ecstatic Dancing session at the community center near where we're now living.

Listening to the music being played, I sensed in myself a change; that is, unlike most of my life when I'd behold something beautiful and be thinking about what comes next, this time I was living in the moment and all I wanted was to appreciate what was.

Returning home, I shared that sentiment with April, and she wondered if Cat Chow might have had a role in gifting me that?...

Earlier in day, in my efforts to recuperate and re-condition, I'd taken a walk to a nearby citrus grove. Along the way, I passed a border collie and appreciated its athleticism, as it went about chasing balls hurled by its owner.

Ini, in all likelihood, had been part border collie (the other part, German shepherd).

Then, as I made my way back home, the border collie went out of its way to drop its ball in front of me and invite me to play. I was still testing positive for the virus, so I kept walking, attempting to give the dog and its owner a wide berth. However, to the consternation of its owner, the dog followed after me and ran in front of me and offered me the ball again; then, it put itself in a prostrate position and waited for me to respond to its entreaty.

I was touched; it felt like this dog knew I needed some canine companionship.

And this dog's act of kindness gave me hope – that, one day, there might be another to touch me as much as Ini.

Every memory of Ini is a blessing, so it's difficult for me to imagine another being comparable to her.

But what greater joy in life is there than companionship?

And perhaps life should engage more than memories?...

On the eve of the year mark of Ini's passing, April asked how I was doing with the COVID infection? I'd been isolating in my room and told her that I thought there was some 'mind-body thing' going on in my chest.

"What do you mean by that?" she asked.

I said sometimes I felt worse than others and thought there was an emotional component to it.

"I think that's well known," she responded. "In Covidland."

"You tried to go back to life, and it knocked you down," she continued. "This is your first Covid experience, and so far, at least, you don't have to go to the hospital."

Yes, I wish I could say I was far from that, but early on, with that shortness of breath and chest discomfort and anxiety, the thought had crossed my mind.

"For some people it's a few days and that's it," she continued. "And for others, it really gets them. And this is how it's getting you."

Yes, I was still in the throes of COVID rebound, an interesting process of mostly awaiting nasal immunity to kick in.

"Yeah, you've got to treat it seriously," she said. "If you don't treat it seriously, and you don't get aggressive about rest, then you're giving it more opportunities to leave you with sequela."

It happens that just before acquiring COVID, I'd reconnected with my Qi Gong master, Master Michael Chou, and members of his group in San Jose offered to help me via 'lightbox' to provide remote healing for my acute COVID.

Master Chou had moved towards sending healing energy like rays of light. In his "Seven Lights of Epidemic Purification" COVID-19 relief treatments, the 1st, 2nd, and 3rd rays of light are for boosting immunity and cleansing the toxins from epidemic infection; the 4th, 5th, 6th, and 7th rays of light are for clearing of soul-related anomalies and adverse vaccine reactions.

A more detailed rendering of those light treatments is as follows:

The 1st Ray of Light
純靛自主光
Pure Indigo Light of Autonomy

The 2nd Ray of Light
金綠光明光
Golden Green Light of Radiance

The 3rd Ray of Light
銀橙安詳光
Silver Orange Light of Serenity

The 4th Ray of Light
銀紅寧靜光
Silver Red Light of Tranquility

The 5th Ray of Light
銀橙安詳光
Silver Orange Light of Serenity

The 6th Ray of Light
純藍自在光
Pure Blue Light of Ease

The 7th Ray of Light
金紫完全開放光
Golden Violet Light of Complete Openness

Usually, when Master Chou's group performed these healings on me, I found myself entering an altered state with the 3rd light, so to suggest that what I needed was serenity and entering a relaxed state.

This last time, though, somehow time stood still at the fourth, fifth, and especially the sixth "blessings", and it struck me, "What if I could be love? What if I could merge with the energy of love in the universe? What if it could be less about me and things outside of love, and I could just merge with love?"

"I would love that," April responded...

April commented how much she missed Ini.

"I feel really proud of us," she said. "I think we were really there for her."

Of course we were, I said. We loved her. She was all that was love. Of course we were there for her.

April had been present for the Qi Gong ceremony with me, and commented about her experiences during the ceremony.

"I found myself remembering times when she was there for me," she said. "My thoughts went back and forth, and I thought about how she was there for me, and I was there for her, and she was there for me. And then, she petted me."

She laughed.

"It was the spirit of Ini," she explained. "It wasn't Ini in the doggie form. It was Ini in the spirit form."

"And then I remembered how it was that she was just so happy," she continued. "Do you remember how she would not stay still anywhere? Like she was bouncy and just so full of happiness and energy? And she would just go round in circles?"

Yes, as a puppy, there wasn't essentially a single photo of her that wasn't a blur.

"And I remember the time that I got lost when we went up to see the falls in the Sierra mountains. And you guys were ahead, and there were several paths, and I didn't know which one you guys took. And she showed up and was like, 'Hey, I'm looking for you.'

"And I remember all the times that she would jump on the bed when you were angry at me, and stand between me and you. She'd be like, 'Knock it off, mom and dad...'"

She reminisced about when Ini became her dog.

"She was very much your dog, in the sense that she would look to you more when we lived in Chamberlain [South Dakota]," she began. "But, then, when we move to DC, she became my dog, because you were busy at work all the time, and I was the one taking her to the park. And she became mine."

That was an awful year, and April, Ini and Cat Chow and living in that hotel was by far the best part of it.

"And Cat Chow would walk with us," she continued. "She hasn't quite walked that way with us anywhere else. She would go all the way into the park and walk around the park with us... All four of us..."

The following morning, April suggested we take a walk.

But I had tested strongly positive for Covid again and didn't want to risk any proximity to her.

"Are you processing Ini's loss?" she asked.

I'd had some thoughts during the night.

April said she'd awoken at about three in the morning, which was about the time we'd made the decision to take Ini to the hospital a year ago to see if there was anything to be done?

Then, she said she woke again at six and recalled that this was about the time we let Ini go.

She said that around this time, Cat Chow had been restless.

"She went outside in the back and then was trying to jump on top of the fence and get over it," she said. "So, I was like, 'I guess Cat Chow really needs out.'

"So, I opened up the gate and she ran out, and then I went after her, and I just followed her. We didn't go very far. I was listening to a couple of songs that I listened to a lot right after Ini died."

She tried to call her mother, who had gone through all of this with us. When her mother didn't answer, she called her sister.

Her sister had made an album with photos of Ini.

"She sent it to us the day after Ini died," April said. "But I just couldn't look at it and then I lost the link. So, she re-sent it.

"And then I was remembering the good times, and I decided to try to put it down.

"I tried to focus on the good memories, and make more space for good memories, and I could put it down, and I didn't have to carry it around... The feelings of guilt and fear... And, 'What if I had done this? Why didn't I do that? Would it have made a difference?' I could put that down. It serves no purpose anymore. I could just put it down and leave it on the ground."

She talked about the conversation she had with her sister.

"She reminded me about something I kept saying after Ini died, but I couldn't actually do, I guess... That what Ini would want is for me to be happy. And that was what she worked hard on all of her life. For me and you to be happy. And Cat Chow. And that was Ini's lifelong wish. To let go of negative things, and look to the positive things.

"I was also thinking of that saying that [Chief] Albert White Hat had framed on the wall next to his seat at the dinner table. It said something to the effect of, 'You are the wolf you feed.' Meaning, there's a positive wolf and a negative wolf, and the more energy you spend on one of those energies, the more you are in that energy.

"So, the time I spend thinking of Ini, I'd like to spend it remembering the fun, loving, amazing stories, rather than the painful stories."

"Do you have any thoughts?" she asked.

I said that Ini was such a positive force, how could you not just think of her with positivity?

She'd asked before if I had been 'processing Ini's loss', and now I shared it: That even that hard time I'd had with seeing Ini in the moment she passed away, now I just think of it like, 'This was a being who wanted to be here and love us in spite of all that unbelievable suffering... What an amazing being! What an amazing, God-gift of a being."

And I love her.

"I love her, too," April said. "How could you not? Ini is love..."

"Oh, and did I tell you what Cat Chow did at three in the morning?" she added, spiritedly. "So, at three in the morning, like when I said, I was up and thinking that this was around the time that we made the decision to take Ini to the hospital, I started crying, even though I had said I was going to try not to do that. I was still doing it a little bit. I was reenacting the day, and I had that moment.

"So, Cat Chow, who had been kind of having the zoomies, so that she wanted to go out, and then she wanted to come in... Well, by now she was on the carpet, and she wasn't even nearby or anything, and I was just in my own little thing, and I started crying.

"And as soon as I started crying, Cat Chow jumped on the couch, and then jumped on the top cushion, and went right behind me.

"And this kind of knocked me out of my crying, and I petted her a little bit, and I was like, 'Ohhh... So sweet.'

"I wonder if that was just purely Cat Chow wanting to make me feel better? Or if Ini told her to do it? Telling her, 'Go comfort mom.'

"Because that was really unexpected. She really did come to me when I was crying. And made herself available for petting. And then, she took me for a walk three hours later."

"Because, you know," she concluded, "Cat Chow talks to the dead..."

ABOUT THE AUTHOR

Michael Yanuck MD PhD is a physician-scientist
whose groundbreaking research at the National Institutes of
Health was the basis for a FDA-approved vaccine for cancer.
Following a traumatic leg injury he returned to medicine. Intent on
caring for the less fortunate, he enlisted in the National Health
Service Corps, worked in urban and rural health centers throughout
the country, then served native peoples in the Indian Health Service.
After three years in the field, he was selected Deputy Director of the
Office of Clinical & Preventive Services at IHS Headquarters.
In 2023 Dr. Yanuck was the recipient of the coveted Science
of Tai Chi & Qigong Award from Harvard University for his
work using BioEnerQi to assist Veterans with problems of
severe traumatic brain injury & neurologic deficits,
chronic pain & opioid dependence, as well as long COVID.
Now, with 30 years' experience in Energy Medicine,
he leads VA efforts to combat the opioid crisis
and advance integrative therapies.

www.ingramcontent.com/pod-product-compliance
Lightning Source LLC
Chambersburg PA
CBHW071346290326
41933CB00041B/2747